Dear Tracy,

To an esteemed professor and good friend of... plastic surgery. With all best wishes.

Peter A. Adamson
July 6, 2011

PRAISE FOR FABULOUS FACES

If your destination is facial enhancement, *Fabulous Faces* reads like a detailed travel guide filled with real stories from real people who took the journey. Lively, witty, and full of practical information, this book is a highly recommended read.

—Donn R. Chatham, M.D.

Past President, American Academy of Facial Plastic and Reconstructive Surgery

Fabulous Faces contains an unparalleled depth of knowledge that single-handedly disproves the old saying about beauty being only skin deep.

—Gabrielle Glaser

Author of *The Nose: A Profile of Sex, Beauty, and Survival*

These patient stories help us all understand that facial plastic surgery affects, not just appearance, but the heart and soul as well. Dr. Adamson has succinctly and honestly provided information that will benefit anyone considering a plastic surgery procedure.

—Wayne F. Larrabee Jr.

President, American Board of Otolaryngology – Head & Neck Surgery

Editor, Archives of Facial Plastic Surgery, American Medical Association

With unflinchingly honest accounts from real people who've undergone facial plastic surgery, *Fabulous Faces* tells it like it really is. This important book explores the human desire to have our outer appearances reflect our inner selves, and gives readers everything they need to know to decide if cosmetic surgery is right for them.

—Shan R. Baker, M.D., F.A.C.S.
Professor and Director, Center for Facial Cosmetic Surgery, University of Michigan

Peter Adamson possesses an almost uncanny understanding of the face and how its changes can affect us. In this book, every dimension of facial aesthetic surgery is explored and presented in clear, accessible writing. *Fabulous Faces* is the ultimate reference book I will be sharing with my patients who are contemplating transformative facial surgery.

—Jim Paupst, M.D.
Toronto Physician and Senior Fellow at Massey College

If you're considering facial plastic surgery, this might be the last book the "old" you ever reads. Dr. Adamson is not only an artist with his technology, but also a master of human nature. He makes the experience of transforming the external into a journey of inner growth.

—Dan Sullivan
Founder, Strategic Coach, Inc.

Fabulous Faces fills a void in patient education for those considering facial plastic surgery. By combining accurate medical information with real-life patient experiences, Dr. Adamson gives readers the knowledge to make informed decisions about potential surgical procedures.

—Ira D. Papel, M.D., F.A.C.S.
President, American Board of Facial Plastic and Reconstructive Surgery and Associate Professor, Johns Hopkins University

Fabulous Faces is a sensitive and intriguing description of what to expect before, during, and following cosmetic surgery. Anyone contemplating a procedure will be both reassured and encouraged.

—Marlene Leeper

Cosmetic surgery patient

Fabulous Faces isn't just about skincare and lifting faces—it's about self-care and lifting spirits. Read this book and look better, feel better, be better.

—Charles Pachter, CM, LLD

Artist, historian and author

FABU
LOUS
FACES

*From Motivation to Transformation
through Plastic Surgery*

FABU
LOUS
FACES

PETER A. ADAMSON, M.D., F.R.C.S.C., F.A.C.S.

ISBN 978-0-9865742-0-7

Publisher's Cataloguing-in-Publication data

Library and Archives Canada Cataloguing in Publication

Adamson, Peter, 1946–
  Fabulous faces : from motivation to transformation through plastic surgery/Peter A. Adamson.

Includes bibliographical references and index.
Issued also in electonic format.
ISBN 978-0-9865742-0-7

  1. Face—Surgery—Popular works.   2. Surgery, Plastic—Popular works.

I. Title.
RD119.5.F33A34 2010   617.5'20592   C2010–904481–9

First Edition

Oslerwood Enterprises
Renaissance Plaza
150 Bloor St. West, Suite M110
Toronto, ON M5S 2X9

Printed in Canada

To all those who have transformed their lives through facial plastic surgery, and to all those seeking the courage to begin their own journeys of self-fulfillment.

CONTENTS

ACKNOWLEDGEMENTS

First and foremost, *Fabulous Faces* is about our patients, how they found their motivation, and how they transformed themselves through facial plastic surgery. I thank them for their trust, and for sharing their stories willingly so they might help others to make this important decision themselves. Our patients have also related how they developed the courage to carry through with their decision. Each patient has taught me something valuable about the human spirit and achieving one's life goals.

My deepest appreciation goes to Michael Lavoie, who explored the world of plastic surgery in order to acquire an intimate knowledge of it. He skillfully interviewed our patients and captured the essence of their stories.

Ana Surghe, our aesthetician, contributed to our chapter on medical Skin Care and continues to have an exceptional ability to make everyone's skin glow.

Susan Morales, R.N., contributed to our chapter on Healing Touch and continues to push the frontiers of wound healing. She has comforted many of our patients after surgery and helped make their transformations much easier.

My teachers from the past provided me the medical, surgical, professional, and ethical foundations to become a facial plastic surgeon. My colleagues today continue to act as my role models and mentors, and constantly spur me to be the best that I can be.

Hundreds of students and residents throughout my career have questioned traditional medical thinking and have spurred the creative thoughts that have helped me to advance our specialty. In particular, my clinical fellows have constantly stimulated my mind and assisted in the care of our patients. They are my living legacy.

At Adamson Associates Cosmetic Facial Surgery, Deborah Doyle encouraged this project from the beginning. Maria Giouzelis continues to use her unique ability to advise our patients and provide them security for a positive experience. Ilya Shkarupin has been a dedicated project manager. Maureen Dennis, R.N., and Joanne Banwell, R.N., have provided the kindest and most expert nursing care for our patients. Shirley Johnstone, R.N., our nurse manager at The Cumberland Clinic, has organized our surgical days and facilitated the collection of our patients' stories. Barry Crane, R.N.A., has dedicated his life to surgical assisting, which has enabled the achievement of the best possible surgical results through his support of me as a surgeon. All of the other Cumberland Clinic staff, including our clinic assistants, recovery room nurses, and anesthesiologists, have worked together seamlessly to create an ideal environment in which to perform procedures for our patients.

The team at Highspot expressed commitment from the beginning that this book would be published. From the outset, their enthusiasm and expert guidance confirmed that this would be a successful project. Carissa Stewart managed our project with clarity and in a timely fashion.

The impetus to write this book came through my association with The Strategic Coach and its founder, Dan Sullivan. To The Coach, I extend my gratitude for helping me create a lifetime of positive energy and providing me the entrepreneurial skills to exceed beyond expectations.

Finally, and most importantly, my family: my children Geoffrey, Heather, and Elizabeth have always been most understanding and accepting of the time required away from them for me to have created a fulfilling professional life. And, of course, their support is a reflection of the administrative, psychological, and spiritual support of my exceptional wife and partner in life, Nora.

With deepest appreciation and gratitude to you all.

YOUR CALLING CARD

Your face is your calling card to the world. Its wondrously complex terrain is uniquely yours. There's no other one just like it. Even when you're silent, your face speaks volumes in the most sophisticated and elegant way. It announces to all, at any given moment, what you are about. It declares your feelings and elicits feelings in others. A smile begets a smile.

The human face has been a source of inspiration for many poets. You pucker your lips for a kiss, and the ghost of Lord Byron goes into rhapsodies: "Her face so fair/Stirr'd with her dream as rose-leaves with the air." Anna Hempstead Branch sees "a web of frail delight." Thomas Campion finds "a garden in her face/Where rose and white lilies grow." French poet and scientist Paul Valéry believed, "We have a spiritual longing to have an outer representation that matches our dreams, visions and moral aspirations."

The face consists of forty-four muscles, which are flat, free-floating, and unattached to bone. As a result, the face is the most mobile and expressive part of the body. California psychologist Paul Ekman and his associates have devised the Facial Action Coding System to catalogue more than 7,000 visually distinguishable facial movements. Ekman sees not roses, lilies, or delightful webs but "a simultaneous contraction of the *incisivus labii superioris* and the *incisivus labii inferioris.*" Even this clinical description rings with its own kind of poetry—the dance of the muscles, the intricate choreography of the face. Love, joy, happiness, curiosity, surprise, confusion, fear, disgust, anger, rage—the face, even the stoniest poker face, announces your feelings.

"Nothing captures our attention like a human face," says Harvard University psychologist Nancy Etcoff, "and nothing rivals the face in communicative power." We talk about faces when expressing our individuality as human beings. Our hearts may be what make us go, but our faces bear the message of our journey.

The story of you is written on your face. But that story sometimes strays into fiction, communicating a false message to the world and keeping the true one under wraps. Faces can mask rather than reveal the person—and the personality—within. People (both men and women) around the world are, in ever-increasing numbers, looking to plastic surgeons to help them discover (or rediscover) their real selves. You may be one of those people.

If you're reading this book—or even browsing it—you're giving plastic surgery some thought. As a facial plastic surgeon, I've had the privilege of studying the beauty of the face and learning its most intricate secrets. My patients have been my teachers, many of them people just like you. This book isn't about me—it's about them and their journeys. Their experiences may help you decide whether you want to follow in their footsteps.

WHAT IS PLASTIC SURGERY?

There's nothing plastic about plastic surgery. The word comes from the Greek *plastikos*, meaning "to mold" or "to give form." The facial plastic surgeon is a sculptor of faces, a practitioner of medicine, and an artist all at the same time. My profession may seem to be relatively new, a late-twentieth-century phenomenon, but it isn't. Plastic surgery is one of the oldest forms of medicine. The first recorded nose reconstructions were performed in India more than 2,500 years ago. Plastic surgery is an ancient art, and the pursuit of beauty is older still. Archaeologists have found traces of red dye that may have been used to adorn faces more than 100,000 years ago.

When people think of plastic surgery for the face—also known as cosmetic facial surgery—they often think of face-lifts and "nose jobs" (the medical term is *rhinoplasty*). There's much more to it than that. In fact, cosmetic facial surgery is a group of procedures carried out singly or in combination, depending on patients' individual needs.

The most common types of cosmetic facial surgery are described below.

Face-lift (Rhytidectomy)

There was a time when the face-lift was simply that. You made incisions around the ears, released the skin of the lower face, lifted it snug, trimmed off the excess, and sewed everything back in place. Now it's different. We don't lift the skin; we lift the underlying tissue so that when the skin is re-draped, there's no tension on it. You don't have that frozen or pulled look.

A face-lift can take away deep wrinkles and folds and remove excess fat at the jawline and neck. It can add definition and contour to the cheeks and chin. It can visibly take years off the face's appearance. However, a face-lift can't completely remove every deep wrinkle or skin fold. It can't add volume to facial tissues. It can't correct skin pigmentation problems. And it can't stop the aging process. It will turn back the hands of time, but the clock will keep ticking.

Eyelid Surgery (Blepharoplasty)

In this procedure, incisions are made in the eyelid creases, following the natural folds to hide the scars. Excess fat, muscle, and loose skin are removed or repositioned.

Eyelid surgery can take away that slightly sinister hooded look from the upper lids and the sagging, pouchy look from the lower lids. If the bags under your eyes look like opera house drapes, a blepharoplasty may be for you. It will diminish, but not entirely eliminate, dark circles. It won't help your crow's feet or correct sagging eyebrows (though other procedures can help).

Nose Job (Rhinoplasty)

Incisions are made under the tip and on the insides of the nostrils (where they aren't visible). Underlying amounts of bone and cartilage are sculpted to make the nose's new shape. The skin is then re-draped over the new frame.

Rhinoplasty can reduce a nose that's too large, narrow a nose that's too wide, straighten a crooked nose, eliminate bumps, reshape the tip, improve the angle between the nose and upper lip, and remove inner obstructions to improve breathing.

Caution

Many other procedures can smoothe wrinkled foreheads, augment chins, correct protruding ears, and tighten sagging necks. Singly or together, these can lead the way to a rekindled life. However, plastic surgery won't guarantee a promotion, bring back a lost love, or turn you into a movie idol.

WHO HAS PLASTIC SURGERY?

Cosmetic facial surgery is no longer the exclusive preserve of socialites, models, and movie stars. More and more ordinary people are having "a little work" done.

- Doreen was in her forties when she faced the exciting—and daunting—prospect of launching a new career. She found herself in the company of smart, ambitious, younger women. "I was forty-seven, and I was competing with twenty-seven," she says. Looking in the mirror, she noticed that her eye makeup was disappearing into the folds around her lids.
- Anne, on the day of her rhinoplasty, said she felt like she was jumping off a cliff. It took her fourteen years to get to the edge of that cliff. She lived for all that time with a nose she thought was "just the ugliest thing in the world," but couldn't bring herself to do anything about it.
- When Christina told her close-knit family that she was considering rhinoplasty, they were furious. Her dad accused her

of turning her back on her strong-featured Italian heritage. Two years later, the wounds are still healing—not from the rhinoplasty, but from the family feud.

– Marguerite went through no end of angst over the money she'd have to spend for her face-lift. Her social conscience nagged and tormented her. She calculated that she could feed an entire village of poor Bolivians with the money she would spend on her face.

– Mary, who came of age in the 1960s, went through a dizzying back and forth over society's obsession with youth. The aging flower child stewed and fretted. It's not what's on the outside that counts, she told herself, it's what's on the inside. However, we live in an age when looks and youth *do* matter.

In this book, more than thirty women—and several men—describe in compelling detail what it's *really* like to go through cosmetic facial surgery. It's a journey that begins long before they get to the operating room. They describe the difficulty in taking the first step: actually giving plastic surgery some serious "this is something I can do" thought. For most, the very idea of "having work" seems preposterous. They move with great deliberation and much soul-searching to another point of view: that plastic surgery isn't about vanity and movie-star looks but is a natural extension of a healthy lifestyle.

ABOUT *FABULOUS FACES*

Fabulous Faces will guide you along the path followed by many patients who decide upon plastic surgery. We begin with the emotional and psychological factors leading people to contemplate plastic surgery:

- initial feelings of dissatisfaction with the face in the mirror
- common fears and myths associated with plastic surgery
- the concept of beauty and its societal influence
- the different views of body image
- events that trigger the decision to pursue plastic surgery

We then move on to finding the right doctor. Finding someone with whom you feel confident, as well as someone you trust, is a big part of the journey. The process includes:

- researching and selecting a doctor, which includes identifying red flags
- learning what to expect during consultation
- determining if you're ready to have plastic surgery

We then take you through the various aspects of plastic surgery from the patient's point of view, such as:

- various levels of skin care, from moisturizers and fillers to laser and Botox®*
- face-lifts—consultation, preparation, surgery, and patient tips
- rhinoplasty—history, psychology, and surgery
- diaries, personal accounts, and stories from patients before, during, and after surgery
- the use of Healing Touch, an alternative method of helping patient recovery
- transformation—patients' reactions to the surgery

We also look at the other faces of plastic surgery: the faces of children with birth defects or serious injuries. Thanks to the support of many of my patients, they're getting a chance to lead normal lives. Every year, I lead a team of doctors to perform restorative surgery on many of these children.

All my patients, in one way or another, tell me that people who undergo cosmetic surgery want their outer appearance to reflect their inner selves. And they want to achieve that with a natural, "unoperated" look. In the words of noted author and critic Camille Paglia, "Good surgery discovers and reveals personality; bad surgery obscures or distorts it." My patients also confirm my belief that facial plastic surgery, whether to change a too-big nose and a too-small chin or to diminish the lines on an aging face, can be—and often is—a life-altering experience.

CHAPTER ONE

To make oneself beautiful is a universal instinct.

– Max Beerbohm, critic and essayist

THE FACE IN THE MIRROR

Marie, Linda, and Kimberly are three of my patients. They could also be your next-door neighbors. One is a retired teacher, one is a busy executive, and one is a retired nurse. They're all in their mid-fifties. Their children have grown up and left home. By any way you want to measure it, they're regular people.

Allow me to introduce them.

MARIE

Marie is a fifty-five-year-old retired teacher who loved her job. A few years ago, she was on yard duty, having one of those glad-to-be-alive days. Then an eight-year-old approached her and asked a life-changing question: "Why are you mad?"

The child saw anger in Marie's face. But she wasn't angry. Her face was betraying her. With the arrival of menopause and decreased production of estrogen, she'd begun to lose the soft features of her face and gentle female allure. Gauntness had crept in. The small lines between her nose and mouth and across her forehead were beginning to look like furrows. Overall, her face was becoming more masculine. It's one of nature's cruel tricks: as women age, their faces can begin to look less feminine.

Marie is not only well-adjusted and emotionally stable but also in great shape. She runs half-marathons. But her aging face was at odds with this reality. Marie saw an older woman with droopy eyes and a matching neck looking back at her in the mirror. Marie started wearing turtlenecks.

Marie thought about a face-lift but pushed the idea to the back of her mind. "It's not your looks—it's your personality and your character that are important," she told herself. But still, the child's question wouldn't go away.

LINDA

Linda manages a human resources department in a large company. As with most executives, her appearance is important. So it was unsettling when co-workers approached her and asked in modulated, consoling voices if she was okay. They would say, "You look sad," or "You look so tired." One colleague, not knowing her age, ventured that she must be getting ready for retirement. She was fifty-one.

Linda's problem was an aging face—droopy lower eyes, a forehead that seemed permanently wrinkled, and a jowly look beneath the chin. It ran counter to her healthy, active lifestyle.

Linda approached cosmetic facial surgery in a very matter-of-fact way, but that soon changed. "It started as a very superficial thing," she says, "but as I went through it, it became a very emotional and spiritual process. It became a life-transforming experience that, in the end, had nothing to do with my face."

KIMBERLY

Kimberly is a fifty-eight-year-old retired nurse and a kind, sensitive woman. She leads a contented life today, but for many years, that wasn't the case. She's naturally shy and introverted in that head-down way that characterizes people who are supremely self-conscious. When she walked down the street, she looked at the sidewalk, avoiding strangers' stares.

As a child, Kim had gone over the handlebars of her bike and broken her nose. It hadn't healed well. "It was bent, right in the center," she says. "It looked like I was walking down the street sideways." She endured schoolyard taunts. Callous boys yelled, "You're so ugly," or, turning a cartoon character into a nasty weapon, addressed her as "Captain Hook." Kim carried the awareness and emotional pain of those taunts through much of her life.

Kimberly's crooked nose turned her into a shrinking violet. As a teenager, she wanted to be a lawyer and dreamed of becoming a judge. But the thought of being in a courtroom, the center of attention, invariably filled her with dread and she pushed the dream away. Instead, Kim turned to nursing because she thought people would be more understanding. But even that was a trial.

Kim pressed on in her head-down way, eventually getting married and raising children. She was too busy running her household and taking care of her family to even think about plastic surgery. But her self-esteem took a terrible beating, and her marriage eventually failed. She says, "He had very bad eyesight, and I used to think, 'Maybe he loves me because he can't see me that well.'"

When her kids grew up and moved away, Kim settled quietly into her empty nest. "The only place I felt comfortable was in the privacy of my own home," she says. "But even there, whenever I looked in a mirror to style my hair or apply makeup, I was reminded of my defect."

Note that Kim doesn't have a nose; she has a "defect." This is the very definition of self-consciousness.

Over the years, Kim soldiered on. Then she faced a series of events that are all-too-familiar among middle-aged women: the mammogram, discovery of a lump, biopsy, diagnosis, followed by tears, surgery, chemo, hair loss, and finally remission. Kim now had that special view of the world accessible only to those who have come face to face with breast cancer. Foremost in her mind was the realization that she'd survived and that life is both fragile and finite.

After recovery, Kim decided to do something just for herself—for her mental health, as she put it. At our first consultation, she said, "I know I'll never be a *Vogue* model. I don't care. I just want to blend in."

Two Sides of Plastic Surgery

Marie, Linda, and Kimberly represent the two sides of my practice:
  – Patients with contour problems—they don't like something about their faces

– Patients seeking rejuvenation—they don't like what their faces have become

In both cases, cosmetic surgery can fill an emotional or psychological gap. Having protruding ears set back, a chin augmented, or a nose reduced enables them (in their own minds) to move from the unattractive or "not normal" group to a group in which they can consider themselves "normal." The French poet Paul Valery once said, "We have a spiritual longing to have an outer representation that matches our dreams, visions and moral aspirations."

A patient with a contour problem has been aware of it since puberty or even early childhood. That awareness can be devastating. A child with protruding ears or crooked nose is very likely to be called hurtful names in the schoolyard, and bullied kids are more likely (40 percent more likely, according to one study) to develop emotional problems than other children.

An aging face problem can develop slowly over the years or hit you quite suddenly. You can look into the mirror one morning and feel as though you're staring into the future. Your reflection isn't the "you" as you imagine yourself but an older version of you—somebody more like one of your parents, an older sibling, or a stern older relative you see only at family reunions. And that may make you feel uncomfortable and perhaps disappointed as well.

You've followed all the rules—eating the right food, exercising, protecting yourself with sunblock—but to no avail. It's enough to make you angry. You have an "angry face" when you're not angry, and *that* makes you angry. Life is so complicated.

People who are courageous enough to undergo cosmetic surgery want their outer appearances to reflect their inner selves. Most of my patients say that they want to look natural. They don't want people to know that they've had things done. They just want to look better. As Kim says, it's not about standing out—it's about blending in. That's not a bad goal. Let's find out how to achieve it.

CHAPTER TWO

Fortis fortuna adiuvat.
(Fortune favors the brave.)

— *Terence,* playwright

THE COURAGE FACTOR

MARIE: ONE WOMAN'S FEAR

Marie first set foot in a plastic surgeon's clinic when she was in her late thirties. She was worried about her eyes. The upper lids had started getting that hooded look that can add years to the appearance of a face. The lower lids were also sagging.

Before coming to me, Marie made an appointment at a well-known plastic surgery clinic. She wasn't sure she was doing the right thing. She never considered herself the plastic surgery type. "I was so nervous," she recalls. "I thought, 'What am I doing?' I wondered what my friends would think."

Marie arrived in a state of anxiety. She opened the door to an unwelcome sight: a crowded waiting room. Women looked up from their magazines and stared. "Can I help you?" the receptionist asked.

Marie felt a jolt of panic. "Sorry, I've made a mistake," she told the startled receptionist. "This isn't for me." She turned and fled. It would take her twenty years to return.

FACING YOUR FEARS

No one decides to get plastic surgery on a whim. Going for a surgical solution to a problem with an aging face or a crooked nose is the polar opposite of making an impulse purchase. Most people think about it for months and proceed only with great caution and much skepticism. Some take years or even decades to decide.

The most common obstacle for someone considering plastic surgery is the fear of an unfavorable result. It's not the fear that you won't get everything you want, but the chilling dread of a Titanic-level disaster. You've heard the stories: Your Pilates instructor's niece had her nose done and can now only breathe through her mouth. Or, as Sylvia (who has a house in Florida) says, "Down there, every second woman looks like she can't close her mouth."

Many people are afraid of the anesthetic. It's a pretty scary prospect to have yourself voluntarily knocked out with drugs while a machine helps you breathe for two or three hours. What if you died on the operating table? What would people say? Dire warnings from the Old Testament about vanity swirl in your head. Your friend's mother had a face-lift and left instructions that, if the worst happened, she should tell everyone that her mother was having a hysterectomy.

Based on these fears, you may think that only a fool would have cosmetic surgery. But only a fool would forge ahead unaware of the risks. And you're not a fool. By reading this book, you're trying to educate yourself and determine what's in your own best interests.

The courageous person knows the risks, understands what's in store, and takes decisive and, sometimes, life-altering action. It takes real courage to go ahead with cosmetic facial surgery, but that courage has little to do with your initial fears. Let's dispel those fears or at least put them in perspective.

'Tisn't life that matters!
'Tis the courage you bring to it.

— *Sir Hugh Walpole*, author

Disasters in cosmetic surgery are quite rare. The overall satisfaction rate is very good, and it's even higher when the surgeon takes a conservative, less-is-more approach. Good cosmetic surgery should never announce itself. The ultimate test is this: You *feel* better because you *look* better. You know you look better because people tell you so—but they can't put their finger on exactly what it is about you that's changed. It's that subtle. It's not about standing out; it's about blending in.

In very rare cases, an adverse reaction to anesthesia could result in a heart attack or stroke. There are other risks as well, which we'll go into later. Much care is taken in advance to identify potential risk factors. These include a preoperative screening process, questions about your medical history, X-rays, blood tests, and a medical examination performed by your family doctor. A normal, healthy individual has little to fear from anesthesia or complications during surgery.

It all comes down to having the information you need to make the best decision for yourself. You don't really *want* an operation. But you may be willing to *endure* one to get from where you are to where you want to be.

And another thing: We've been talking about surgery, but there are also many nonsurgical, noninvasive treatments that you can have (see Chapter 7). These usually have minimal or no side effects or downtime.

FANTASY MEETS REALITY

Natasha

Natasha is a soft-spoken English woman with a warm, empathetic personal style. She's also a psychiatrist. She's never thought of herself as pretty, but friends and family had always said she had a mobile, sympathetic face. Still, by the time she turned fifty, Natasha found herself spending more and more time at the mirror, wistfully studying her reflection.

She would place her fingertips on her cheeks and push her face back into a younger, trimmer, less saggy position. She'd briefly lament the passage of time, indulge in some vague yearnings for a fountain of youth, and get on with her day. Call it the opposite of preening. Cosmetic surgery wasn't on Natasha's to-do list. She wasn't even considering it—or so she thought at the time. After her surgery, she said, "I was thinking about it, but I wasn't aware I was thinking about it."

Natasha isn't alone. If you're like her, you're thinking about plastic surgery, but you're not *really* thinking about it. The idea floats around in the subconscious. You let it out to play every so often but quickly call it home. A persistent, nagging voice in the back of your mind tells you that it's somehow *wrong*. Natasha feared "a kind of Godly judgment on my vanity." The result would be divine payback—a bolt of lightning that reduces you to nothing but a pair of shoes and a small pile of ashes.

The very idea of cosmetic surgery at first seems preposterous. It's just a fantasy, like moving to Venice and becoming a gondolier. Face-lifts and nose jobs are something that *other* people get—the pampered, the self-absorbed, famous people, neurotics, and those occupying a rarefied place far outside the mainstream.

That's not you. You're down-to-earth, a realist living in the real world. Cosmetic surgery is a pipe dream. You push the thought out of your mind and turn to other matters.

But just a minute! This isn't about turning you into something false. It's not as if you want a Hollywood face with a button Barbie nose and pouty Angelina lips. You just want to be *you*, but a refreshed version of you, a younger you. Like it or not, we live in a time and place that values youth and imposes unfair penalties on age.

Mary-Anne

Mary-Anne was driven by the same motivation. When she turned fifty, she wanted to have her face and eyes done. She's an accountant with a busy big-city practice. The first sign of trouble came not from friends, family, or business associates but from restaurant maître d's who began seating her next to the kitchen door. Mary-Anne began to get angry with society. She was becoming one of the invisible people.

Marie

Marie, who came of age with the flower children in the sixties, considers herself all-natural. Like Mary-Anne, she came up against the same table-at-the-back problem. Marie sees it as age-ism and believes that it's a reality of our times that people need to look young, fit, and healthy.

Liz

Liz, a media marketer, says, "I work in a very young industry, and my success almost totally depends on my ability to communicate with my customers. It's a lot easier when they relate to me more as an older colleague than as a friend of their mothers."

Natasha, Mary-Anne, Marie, and Liz have one thing in common: Their outer appearances were at odds with their inner spirits. They all took the plunge. You may not be ready to do the same. But you've moved along. You've given yourself permission to entertain the thought of cosmetic surgery. It's no longer locked away in the fantasy box with the gondolier's hat. This is something that you could possibly, perhaps consider doing one day. But so far, you've told no one. What's your next step?

If you're like most of my patients, you'll go into fact-finding mode, spending hours on the Internet looking for explanations of surgical procedures, finding the names of doctors, and browsing cosmetic surgery chat rooms. This goes a long way toward normalizing the whole process, transforming it from something that *they* do to something that *you* could do.

Cosmetic surgery is now a distinct possibility. You're not committed to it yet. But it's definitely on your radar. What's next?

TO TELL OR NOT TO TELL

But now comes another moment of truth. You've been putting it off, but you can't any longer—not if you're serious. This is where the courage kicks in. You have to tell someone. I'm not saying you have to "go public." You don't have to rent a billboard, buy an ad in the paper, or shout it from the rooftops. This particular journey is private and personal, one that you're taking for yourself alone.

James

James writes, "As I reflect back, one main theme jumps up continually, and that is that you should have the surgery for one person's satisfaction, and only one person's satisfaction, and that person is yourself. You're setting yourself up for failure otherwise."

James makes an important point. If your reason for proceeding is to please someone else, you should reconsider the whole trip. This isn't for you. That said, you shouldn't proceed solo. Somebody else needs to come on board. It could be your closest friend, the one who, as one poet said, "knows the song of your soul and sings it back to you when you've forgotten the words." It could also be a family member, a son or daughter, or a brother or sister. And who else? How about the person next to you in bed, your beloved, snoring spouse?

This is where it gets tricky, especially if you're a woman. It takes nerve and a touch of bravery. Tell a husband over breakfast that you're thinking of getting a face-lift, and he's likely to drop his toast. He may also think you've taken leave of your senses. Remember, while you've been thinking about your face, he's probably been thinking about sports or the newspaper he's reading. And if you're a man, your partner is even less likely to think your appearance is of any concern to you.

Arpi

That's pretty much how it went with Arpi. She comes from a very direct, no-nonsense family in which everyone says exactly what's on their minds. She sat her husband down, told him she wanted a smaller nose, and filled him in on her plans for Operation Rhinoplasty. He told her she was nuts—she was beautiful.

But you can see the husband's dilemma. Either he thinks you're beautiful and don't need cosmetic surgery, or he thinks you're looking a little rough around the edges and that a face-lift or nose job would be a good idea.

In either case, he's likely to look around wildly for the exit. His survival instinct will kick in. He's been through this before— the "Do I look fat in this dress?" question—and realizes there's only one answer: No. You don't need it. You're perfect just as you are.

Marie

Marie considered an end run around involving her spouse. Her problem lay in her husband's wallet. He keeps a snapshot of her, one taken years ago when she was in the full flush of youthful beauty. He likes to look at it and tell her that she still looks eighteen. It's sweet, and she loves him for it. But it really isn't helpful when you're considering a face-lift. That left Marie thinking, "Oh, I don't want to involve him. He's going to be so worried."

Marie actually planned to go ahead with the procedure and spend three or four days afterward in a hotel room. She wisely reconsidered and told her husband. "He practically had a heart attack," she recalls. But they talked it through. He got on board when it became apparent that his wife really wanted to pursue this goal.

Telling Friends and Family

Many people try to keep the whole thing a secret from spouses, family, and friends until the deed is done. They almost always reconsider. I'm sometimes asked for surgery dates that coincide with a spouse being away on a business trip. Here's my advice: Don't have your face-lift in January because Harry will be in Singapore. Have it when Harry's at home and available to hold your hand. If he's like most husbands, he'll want to.

Sons and daughters are another matter. They can be difficult. Doreen decided to have a face-lift at the age of sixty-four. Facing the surgery was a lot easier than facing her son and two daughters. "They ganged up on me," she says. "They told me, 'We don't want you to do this. You're healthy. You should be happy. What are you looking for?'"

Adult children can be anxious and judgmental. They don't want Mom to change. They may be all grown up with families of their own, but they're still children around you. In my experience, children who deliver the "What can you be thinking?" speech almost always come around when they realize that the parent is going ahead no matter what. One thing you can do in such circumstances is to gently remind children or spouses that you've often supported them in decisions you may not have agreed with and that now you would like—and expect—them to support you.

That's what happened with Doreen. Eventually she told her children, "Hey, like it or not, it's my decision and I'm going to do it." With that, the fierce opposition died down. After the surgery, Doreen's son collected her and took her home. "I looked like the Cheshire cat," she says. "I was all smiles because I'd done it."

But what about others, such as your friends and co-workers? The "What will people think?" worry often turns out to be misplaced. The people you feel you need to tell are usually fine with it. Natasha told three friends. "The friends I find most valuable," she says, "are the non-judgmental ones."

COSMETIC SURGERY MYTHS

Many fears are based on what we don't know, as well as what we think we know. Many people have preconceived notions about cosmetic surgery. Their assumptions are based on myths and hearsay. Knowing the facts can clear up most misconceptions and dispel their fears at the same time.

Myth: Only rich people have cosmetic surgery

Plastic surgery used to be the preserve of movie stars, models, and the very wealthy. They'd visit exclusive clinics in New York or Los Angeles for a face-lift or rhinoplasty.

In the fifties and early sixties, the trendy thing was the "nose bob." Everyone who was anyone wanted a pert little nose, also known as the Debbie Reynolds or Judy Garland look. Some procedures were even named for the doctors who performed them. Manhattan surgeon Irving Goldman developed a rhinoplasty technique that produced a small nose with a slightly upturned tip. Having the "Goldman tip" was instantly identifiable and a sure sign that you were part of the *in* crowd. These changes had nothing to do with your personality or character. In fact, they often disguised the real you.

Today, face-lifts and rhinoplasties are meant to achieve the opposite result. They reveal rather than disguise character and aren't supposed to announce themselves. It's not about standing out; it's about blending in.

Some skeptics believe that people have cosmetic surgery to change themselves into something they're not. The reality is quite the opposite. Most people who have cosmetic facial surgery are driven by a desire to discover and reveal who they really are. It's not about looking for the "new me." It's about finding the "real me." The rewards of that discovery can be considerable. A face refreshed by cosmetic surgery, or a facial contour problem resolved once and for all, can and often does generate a new spark of vitality.

When it's done "under the radar," the changes are both dramatic and subtle. You could walk past people like Marie or Kimberly—or meet them face-to-face—and never suspect that they had "had work." They look great, but they don't look like they've had anything done. The "done look" is the last thing they want.

These types of people also represent the new face of cosmetic surgery in North America. They're ordinary people and definitely not part of the entertainment or fashion industry elite. In 2005, the American Society of Plastic Surgeons (ASPS) surveyed people considering plastic surgery within the next two years. Seventy-one percent of respondents reported an average annual household income of $60,000 or less, and 30 percent earned less than $30,000. Cosmetic surgery is no longer just for the rich.

Myth: Only vain people have cosmetic surgery

We all want to look our best—and most of us are deeply conflicted about it. List the pros and cons of having cosmetic surgery, and the word "vanity" invariably appears on the "con" side.

The truly vain person's entire sense of self-worth revolves around his or her appearance. You may know such people. They're often consumed by a desire for more of everything. They're beautiful, but not beautiful enough. They have an unrealistic sense of entitlement and are invariably frustrated when things don't go their way. Does that sound like you? Probably not.

You're concerned about your aging face but not consumed by it. Unlike the truly vain person, you stew and fret about what others may think. It isn't so much about vanity as it's about being seen as vain. Harvard psychologist Nancy Etcoff says in her book *Survival of the Prettiest* that our beauty, as others judge it, isn't linked strongly to self-esteem. While self-image is determined by how others see us, self-esteem is determined by how we see ourselves. Etcoff quotes Eleanor Roosevelt, who was sensitive about her distinctive but not classically beautiful looks, as saying, "No one can make you feel inferior without your consent."

There's something more primal about it. We're hardwired to both survive and reproduce. A sagging jowly face, hooded eyelids, or a drooping nasal tip are unwelcome signs of age and mortality. We look for ways to turn back the hands of time. Beyond that, we're all players in the reproductive sweepstakes. Wanting to appear sexually attractive is a signal of health and vitality—and an innate desire.

In my opinion, it isn't as much about vanity as it's about having the courage to take a big, life-altering step to do something for yourself. This is the main source of conflict. It's rare to meet a cosmetic surgery patient who hasn't thought long and hard about the process.

Sarah is a successful, independent, forty-year-old single woman with a career as a medical research co-ordinator. Until she had it fixed, she had a nose that she had hated since puberty. It was big and crooked. For years, she thought about rhinoplasty, even made plans for it, but always backed away. She kept telling herself that wanting to change her nose was simply a reflection of her lack of self-worth.

Marguerite had doubts about what her family and friends would think. Her daughter was aghast. Before the surgery, when the subject came up among friends, one said that Marguerite would never do such a thing. She was too *au naturel* for that. Facing that kind of skepticism, incredulity, and outright opposition from those closest to you can be very difficult.

When Christina was in her twenties, she raised the subject of rhinoplasty with her family. "Get your head on straight," her dad told her. Her family laid a huge guilt trip on her, telling her that wanting to change the contour of her nose was a sign of weakness on her part. They played the ethnicity card, accusing her of turning her back on her strong-featured Italian heritage. Years later, there are still some issues about it within the family, but they're being resolved.

Doreen, a widow in her sixties, encountered opposition from her grown children and some work colleagues. Her children told her she was being vain, while her co-workers said that she looked fine as she was and didn't need it. Doreen says there was also an underlying suspicion that she was out to get a man. "People don't always understand you," she says. "They presume that I'm either looking for a male friend or have some other reason beyond just wanting to do it for myself, so I had to start saying, 'Look, I want this just for me, just for myself. When I look in the mirror, I want these wrinkles to be gone.'"

Once the perception of vanity takes hold, it's often accompanied by guilt. Some guilt comes from within, but much of it is imposed by others' judgments. You're doing something just for yourself—not for your spouse or your children—and you feel bad about it or others make you feel bad about it. This can be a nerve-racking experience and very difficult to overcome. The people nearest and dearest to you can cause you to doubt yourself. But in the end, your family and true friends will come around. As financier and statesman Bernard Baruch once said, "Those who matter don't mind, and those who mind don't matter."

Some believe that the media encourages people to have cosmetic surgery. It's the "in thing" to do. Television and entertainment magazines are full of stories, some true and some pure nonsense, about aging celebrities who have had work done. I don't buy it. I think people are primarily driven by their own desire to look their best.

I also see evidence in my patients that any lingering sense of guilt goes away after surgery. When people feel better about themselves, they contribute more to society. They do more for others. If you're better able to realize your own expectations in life, you're likely to do more for others.

Generally, people who undergo cosmetic surgery feel like outsiders and just want to be part of the "normal" group. They aren't looking to be better than everyone else or trying to live forever. They just want to be part of the crowd. It's not about vanity; it's about courage.

Myth: Only women have cosmetic surgery

Many men have had cosmetic surgery, including face-lifts, rhinoplasties, forehead lifts, eyelid surgery, laser skin resurfacing, and fillers. This group is growing by about three million men a year. About 16 percent of cosmetic surgery and other cosmetic procedures across North America are done on men.

Matthew, now in his forties, says he's "really struggling with the aging process." Beyond that, he's had a lifelong obsession with his nose, which he thought was too big and had been off-kilter since a childhood playground accident. After his rhinoplasty, he sensed an "internal shift." People seemed more open and friendly to him, not because he looked better (though he did) but because he felt better about himself. They weren't reacting to his rhinoplasty. Few even noticed that he'd had work done. They were reacting to his reaction to the rhinoplasty.

Gordon had a similar experience. During his thirty-seven years with a utility company, he paid little attention to his appearance. He retired at age fifty-five and began thinking about improving his self-respect and self-confidence. Gordon had a face-lift and noticed a change in himself. "It gave me a more positive outlook on life and people reacted to that," he says. "That was nine years ago, and I still don't look a day over fifty-five."

"I didn't do it for anybody else," he adds. "I did it for myself."

These kinds of stories gladden my heart. In my experience, women notice changes in their reactions and the reactions of people around them more readily than men. Men tend to be much more matter-of-fact about their surroundings and about consulting their internal emotional barometers.

Men are also caught up in our youth-oriented times. Fair or not, society rewards youthful looks and imposes penalties on those who don't fit in. For this reason, a growing number of men are having cosmetic surgery so they can hold their own among younger colleagues at work.

Myth: People are never happy with their cosmetic surgery

According to ABC News, more than two-thirds of North American baby boomers say they would consider having cosmetic surgery if they knew it was completely free and safe. So why aren't more people doing it? What's holding them back is fear of the Titanic Effect—the poorly done nose job, the pulled face, or the blank, expressionless look that shouts, "I've had work!"

Anne fretted for fourteen years about her profile. She'd inherited her father's nose, which looked fine on him but didn't, in Anne's opinion, fit well with her delicate features. "Fear of a bad- or unnatural-looking result was the only thing that held me back," she says. After having the surgery, Anne says, "I feel like I've always had this nose. I think it's almost funny how anxious and apprehensive I was about the surgery."

Plastic surgery disasters, though few and far between, always get noticed in the media, especially if they happen to a celebrity. They're usually the result of too much plastic surgery.

Patients tell me all the time that they don't want to look like Joan Rivers, who jokes that her face "has been tucked more times than a bedsheet at the Holiday Inn." To my mind, there are many in the entertainment business whose results are less attractive. And, to her credit, Rivers makes no apologies about her ongoing campaign against the effects of aging. In her book *Men Are Stupid . . . And They Like Big Boobs*, she observes, "In our appearance-centric society, beauty is a huge factor in everyone's professional and emotional success—for good or ill, it's the way things are; accept it or go live under a rock."

One way that surgeons measure success is by the "revision" rate on noses. Those are rhinoplasties that have to be done again because they didn't work the first time. Why noses? Because they're the most difficult to get right. A good cosmetic facial surgeon may have a 10 to 15 percent revision rate on rhinoplasties. But with care and a conservative approach, you can get it down to 5 percent. The aim shouldn't be perfection but improvement.

So the idea that people are never happy with their plastic surgery is false. In my own practice, a study that we did of almost one hundred face-lift and rhinoplasty patients, both men and women, revealed a satisfaction rate of close to 90 percent. These patients viewed plastic surgery not as an indulgence or a luxury, but as a self-image concern that cut to the very heart of social desirability.

Myth: You can always tell when someone has had cosmetic surgery
Turn on *Entertainment Tonight* and play "Spot the Face-lift." Better still, watch the pre-Oscar red-carpet show. Who's had a nose job? Who's a Botox Queen? Are those real? It's a national pastime—harmless fun. But there's a modest downside: Everybody thinks he or she is an expert at detecting cosmetic surgery.

The reality is quite different. You probably see people every day who have had "work" done. You just don't know it.

Mary-Anne: "People who have known me since I was fourteen can't tell."

Natasha: "I look the same as I did before the operation, except people think I'm in my early forties."

Liz: "Nobody knew I had work done. They thought I lost weight."

Doreen wanted to take at least ten days of recovery time after her face-lift but, because of an important conference, returned to work in just one week. "I probably should have waited another couple of days," she says. "I wore my hair forward so they couldn't see any of the scars, and nobody was aware."

Brad had rhinoplasty for a long and crooked nose and an implant for a receding chin. You'd think he'd stand out like Mount Rushmore. He says, "People comment on improvements in my appearance but can't tell why it looks so much better."

People want to alter their appearances but don't want to look as if any alterations have taken place. Make a positive life style change, such as losing weight, quitting smoking, or getting in shape, and you want to shout it from the rooftops. But you want to keep it quiet that you've improved yourself through plastic surgery. On the surface it doesn't seem logical, but it makes perfect sense on a psychological level.

People who have cosmetic surgery see themselves as outside the normal range of where they want to be. They want to move into what they perceive to be the real world of people with normal features. But to make that move, they feel they must remain anonymous. Otherwise, in their minds, they'll be seen as fakes. As soon as you tell someone you've had something done, then it's not the real you. So, people can be very proud of having gone through with cosmetic surgery, as long as they keep it to themselves.

You've taken that first big step: moving cosmetic surgery from the back of your mind to the front. You're no longer in the what-could-I-be-thinking stage. You're now in the this-is-something-I-could-do stage. It's no longer unthinkable; you're thinking about it.

But you're not yet ready to put it on your to-do list. So what's holding you back? It may be your ambivalence about the whole question of beauty. Let's look at that.

CHAPTER THREE

Beauty is a greater recommendation
than any letter of introduction.

— *Aristotle*, philosopher

THE BEAUTY YARDSTICK

DEFINING BEAUTY

Like it or not, the world around us is an ongoing beauty contest. And we're all judges. We don't spend much time in ponderous deliberation. We routinely (and unconsciously) scan strangers' faces, starting with the eyes, and make snap decisions about their looks. We rush to judgment. According to a 1980 psychological study measuring the speed of human visual judgement, it takes place in 150 milliseconds—the blink of an eye, thirty-six times faster than it took you to read this sentence. Everybody does it, and that makes us all unwilling contestants as well as judges. The question is: What are we judging, and how are we being judged?

Measuring the true face of beauty—identifying the features that set a beautiful face apart from a merely attractive one—seems impossible. It's been the preoccupation of the ages. Plato declared that being beautiful was one of the three great wishes of humankind (the other two being good health and riches). Beauty, however it's defined, has always been equated with positive qualities (and ugliness with negative qualities). Sappho said, "What is beautiful is good." Aristotle, for all his wisdom, thought the homely weren't to be trusted. But it's one thing to dress up beauty with qualities and personality traits and another to define it objectively.

The Oxford English Dictionary defines beauty as "excelling in grace of form, charm of coloring, and other qualities which delight the eye and call forth admiration: a. of the human face and figure: b. of other objects."

While researching *Survival of the Prettiest*, which is about the science of beauty, Nancy Etcoff turned to experts in fashion and entertainment for their definitions of beauty. After all, beautiful faces and sexy bodies are their stock in trade. They should know.

Hollywood television mogul Aaron Spelling, creator of *Beverly Hills, 90210*, *Melrose Place*, and *Dynasty*, gave it some thought and then concluded, "I can't define it, but I know it when it walks into the room."

Not much help there. Perhaps the head of a big modeling agency can do better. "It's when someone walks in the door and you almost can't breathe," says Heidi Belmann of the Zoli Agency in New York. "It doesn't happen often. You can feel it rather than see it." In other words, a beautiful face is one that takes your breath away, a face that stops traffic. The fashion and entertainment crowd couldn't describe beauty to Etcoff; they could only describe their reactions to it.

Murad Alam, a plastic surgeon in Massachusetts, encountered the same problem when researching the subject. "We may each know it when we see it, hear it or smell it, but to accurately describe beauty or the features that impart it to a face, song or scent can be daunting," he writes.

Beauty as we feel it is something indescribable: what it is or what it means can never be said.

– *George Santayana*, philosopher

Describing beauty in purely objective terms—quantifying, listing, and labeling its component parts—seems impossible. Where does that leave you? You find yourself browsing through *Peter's Almanac* and come across this irreverent advice: "Always remember that true beauty comes from within—from within bottles, jars, compacts, and tubes."

Perhaps the topic of beauty is better left to lyricists and romance writers. John Keats said, "A thing of beauty is a joy for ever:/ Its loveliness increases; it will never/ Pass into nothingness." Such definitions have the ring of truth. But under the microscope, those definitions invariably deal not with the beautiful object, but the response it evokes.

It seems like a fool's errand. The true face of beauty appears to be the face that you find beautiful, not the face that's beautiful in and of itself. The most beautiful face is the one you fall in love with . . . but did you fall in love just because of the face?

Novelist Henry James once described nineteenth-century novelist George Eliot, whose real name was Mary Anne Evans, as "magnificently ugly" with "a low forehead, dull gray eyes, a vast pendulous nose [and] a huge mouth full of uneven teeth." As harsh and cruel as this seems, he also wrote, "Now in this vast ugliness resides a most powerful beauty which, in a very few minutes, steals forth and charms the mind so that you end as I ended, in falling in love with her." Henry James found her beautiful—not because of her physical appearance, but because of her inner spirit. He got past that initial sixth-of-a-second, blink-of-an-eye assessment and found her beautiful.

You can look at a wrinkled and aged grandparent and see beauty. Mother Teresa's kindness imparted beauty, as did Albert Einstein's wisdom, but neither was a knockout. Where does that leave us? Back at the great truth: Beauty is in the eye of the beholder.

MEASURING BEAUTY

However, you may be surprised to know that our ideas of beauty can be objectively measured. It involves mathematical precision. Beauty has its own metes and bounds, which are calculated in fractions of a millimeter. The subtle and abstract concept of beauty can be—and is—subject to the cold stare of science.

David Perrett measures how we recognize facial attributes that give cues to attractiveness and health, and quantifies these with skill and exactitude. A cognitive psychologist at the University of St. Andrews in Scotland, he has made it his life's work to understand what makes faces attractive.

Perrett runs a "perception lab" with a worldwide reputation as a leading center for the study of beauty. He uses a computerized morphing system that can take any face and endlessly adjust its features. Then he gets opinions on his images. It's like an ongoing Gallup Poll of beauty, a focus group for faces. Volunteers rate faces according to how beautiful they find them. Perrett then turns people's reactions to the images into an objective assessment of our perceptions of beauty.

Perrett's findings are remarkable. His research suggests that a conventionally attractive female face becomes beautiful if it has just one or two characteristics that fall outside of what we consider to be the average range. It doesn't take much to make the transformation. Perrett says that the most attractive female faces stand out because they have one or more of the following features:

- thin jaws and small chin
- large, widely spaced eyes
- small nose
- high cheekbones
- short distances between mouth and chin
- short upper lips

These are the very features that play up the ways in which women's faces differ from men's faces. Imagine the man of your dreams. Is he thin-jawed, big-eyed, and short-nosed? Probably

not. These are the defining features of female beauty. Male faces are judged most attractive by the following features:
- rectangular faces
- prominent chins
- deep-set eyes
- heavy brows
- lustrous, abundant hair

The classically beautiful face has always been defined in terms of symmetry and ratios. The early Greeks had an extensive catalogue of what worked and what didn't in a human face. The sculptor Phidias used a mathematical formula called the golden ratio (1:1.618). It's the division of a line so that the relation of the smaller section to the larger is the same as the relation of the larger to the whole. This ratio appears throughout nature and is easily found in our own bodies. In classically beautiful people, the mouth is 1.6 times wider than the width of the nose. Each finger joint is about 1.6 times the length of the next. Nancy Etcoff says that, with a protractor and set of calipers, the golden ratio can be found everywhere—in shells, flower petals, architectural forms, and faces.

There's some argument as to whether the golden ratio really works. The proportions can be easily found in the faces of fashion models. Orthodontist Stephen Marquardt mapped the faces of ten models and found the magic ratio everywhere, even in the comparative sizes of their teeth. Many consider it an unimportant fluke, while others say that it's a legitimate way to measure beauty.

Beyond ratios (and concern about whether your eyes are in balance with your nose), there's another way of objectively measuring beauty. That lies in symmetry, the duplication of a feature on each side of a line—eyes that match precisely, nostrils that look like mirror images, and so on. Symmetry creates facial harmony. In this area, most of us are at some disadvantage. An estimated 85 percent of human faces aren't symmetrical. That means the other 15 percent are perfectly symmetrical. In pure survival-of-the-fittest evolutionary terms, the symmetrical face advertises sexual health, making that face's bearer a good candidate for reproduction. The asymmetrical face can carry the opposite message. It used to be associated with illness.

THE CONCEPT OF "AVERAGENESS"

The biology of beauty doesn't stop there. It also explores the idea of *averageness* as a marker for beauty. This may seem contradictory. Beautiful? No, just average. We're talking about faces that are average in shape. When you make composite pictures of faces, superimposing one on top of another, something strange happens. The face invariably begins to look better. This was first discovered in the 1870s by Sir Francis Galton, Charles Darwin's eccentric half-cousin. Galton began assembling composite images of English criminals. In picture after picture, the men had the appearance of those who had led rough and ruthless lives. But as more faces were added, one superimposed on another, a strange thing happened. The composite image, though blurry, began to look more benign.

A century later, California anthropologist Donald Symons took the idea of averageness a step further. When looking at slides of extraordinarily beautiful people, he noticed that each was somehow imperfect—a too-long upper lip, or a too-prominent nose. He wondered what he was using as a basis of comparison and decided that it was his own mental image of average beauty. He concluded that human facial beauty is average and that our brains collect images of people and turn them into composites (as Galton did). To him, beauty became the departure from average in at least one feature. Sexual psychologist Havelock Ellis wrote that "the absence of flaw in beauty is itself a flaw."

I'm tired of all this nonsense about beauty being only skin-deep. That's deep enough. What do you want—an adorable pancreas?

– Jean Kerr, author

THE CULTURE OF BEAUTY

As contestants in the Great Beauty Contest, we all have to take our chances. But how do we stack up as judges? We all have built-in beauty detectors, which seem to be wired the same way worldwide. From 1989 to 1990, psychologist David Buss conducted a survey across six continents, interviewing people of all ages from thirty-seven different cultures about their preferences in a long-term partner. In every case, good looks and healthy bodies were high on the list. In many cases, beauty received higher marks than personality traits such as dependability, emotional stability, and maturity.

Beyond that, the results seemed to dispute claims by Western feminists—such as Naomi Wolf, author of *The Beauty Myth*—that true, objectively defined beauty doesn't exist. Wolf asserted that much of it is cooked up by Madison Avenue advertising men to keep women in an ornate but subservient place, and that though the pursuit of beauty is a legitimate part of our lives, it can be dangerous when taken to extremes of thinness and youthfulness.

Nevertheless, humankind has been obsessed with beauty throughout history. There are many examples:

- Archaeologists digging at sites in southern Africa up to 120,000 years old have found traces of red ocher that some believe may have been used to paint the face and body.
- The ancient Egyptians rouged their lips and cheeks, stained their nails, and lined their eyes with kohl, a powder made of crushed antimony and burnt almonds. Displayed in the British Museum is an Egyptian woman's toilet chest that contains an ivory comb, a bronze cosmetic dish, vases for skin salves, a pumice stone, and a pair of leather sandals. It's believed to be almost 3,600 years old.
- In ancient Greece, cosmetics was a booming cottage industry. Every town had its perfume merchants selling various scents in small ceramic pots similar to the jars sold in Athens today.
- In Japan, about a thousand years ago, kimonos had an accessory: a small lacquer case that hung from a clasp and contained perfume. This inspired the design of the container for today's Opium brand of perfume.

So it's not just a modern idea, and it's not going away. Etcoff says, "We can create a big bonfire with every issue of *Vogue*, *GQ*, and *Details*, every image of Kate Moss, Naomi Campbell, and Cindy Crawford, and still, images of youthful, perfect bodies would take shape in our heads and create a desire to have them."

The love of beauty is innate, affecting people of all cultures. The beauty template also seems to be similar across cultures. When shown pictures of different faces, Japanese and Scottish students found the same ones attractive.

CHILDREN AND BEAUTY

You might think that our beauty detectors don't kick in until puberty, when we begin considering romantic relationships and worrying about how our looks measure up. In fact, we're tuned in at a much earlier age. "Many people have an idyllic conception of childhood as a time when beauty doesn't matter," says Etcoff. "Listen to children taunt and tease each other in the schoolyard—'shrimp,' 'squirt,' 'four-eyes,' 'fatso'—to quickly disabuse yourself of that notion." Children, says Etcoff, gravitate to beauty.

Their judgments about beauty are influenced by their surroundings, their parents, their friends, and cultural trends. But there's a deeper influence that seems to be hardwired into all of us. Psychologist Judith Langlois gathered pictures of faces and had adults rate them for beauty. When she showed the pictures to three- and six-month-old infants, they gazed longer at the attractive faces. This experiment worked for a variety of male and female faces of different ages and races. The babies spent more time looking at the images judged to be attractive. Langlois believes we're born with pre-programmed beauty detectors. Others believe the preferences are "imprinted" on infant brains and that a learning process occurs rapidly without an obvious linguistic component.

THE PSYCHOLOGY OF BEAUTY

Like it or not, looks matter. They confer rewards on the beautiful and impose penalties on the plain. Consider some recent findings by psychologists:

- College students were shown pictures of attractive and unattractive women, then asked to select who they would do one of the following for:
  - help move furniture
  - loan money
  - donate blood
  - donate a kidney
  - swim a mile to rescue
  - save from a burning building
  - fall on a live grenade

Men most often opted to perform the riskiest acts for the beautiful women (except when it came to loaning them money).

- A coin was left in a telephone booth. A woman, either pretty or plain, approached and asked the occupant if her coin was there. Eighty-seven percent returned the coin to the pretty woman, while only 64 percent returned the coin to the plain one.
- Tall is better than short. Asked to approach a stranger and stop when they feel uncomfortable, people will stop almost two feet away from a tall person but less than a foot away

from a short one. The tall gain more personal territory by their height alone.

- Good-looking people have a sense of entitlement. A psychologist set up a test in which he brought subjects in for interviews and, by pre-arrangement, was interrupted by a colleague and left the room. Attractive people waited an average of three minutes and twenty seconds before demanding attention. The unattractive waited an average of nine minutes.
- Tall, square-jawed West Point graduates are more likely to achieve high military rank than shorter, less imposing classmates.
- Pretty high-school girls are ten times more likely to marry than plainer classmates.

If you believe psychologists, beautiful people get better grades, have better jobs, earn more money, receive better service, and enjoy better sex lives. They're even more successful as criminals. A 1997 study reported that beautiful lawbreakers are more likely to be acquitted or receive light sentences—except for fraud. Judges and juries tend to deal more harshly with physically attractive swindlers and con artists than with plainer ones (who presumably don't rely on their looks to carry out their crimes).

BEAUTY AND GENETICS

We like to think we live in an age when looks don't matter. We want to believe that it's not what you are on the outside, but what you are on the inside that counts. But the hard truth is that we can't fight our genetic makeup. We have descended from tribal "survival of the fittest" societies in which the weak died young. Survival was directly linked with reproductive ability. Those things are no longer inextricably linked in our world today, but our genes don't know that.

Evolutionary psychologists believe that attractive faces advertise good genes, which want to be passed on. An attractive face is a health certificate proclaiming an individual's value as a mate. A healthy appearance suggests fertility and reproductive capacity.

Interestingly, psychologists have found that women's sexual response to attractive men actually increases, with no conscious effort on their part, during the fertile period of their menstrual cycles. At other times, that attraction lessens and women have a soft spot for men with more feminine or "baby-faced" features. In studies, women associated this with warmth, honesty, and a willingness to invest in offspring.

In either case, the first drive of human beings is to survive, and part of that is reproduction. That's why sex is so important and why fashion and beauty become important. They're all related to sex.

Most people who want rhinoplasty started to dislike their noses at puberty, when it came time to be accepted by the opposite sex. Darwinian evolutionary thinkers would say that if we don't want to die, and one of our primal drives is to survive, then certainly we can see by looking at our own skin that we are getting old and will die. We're on that route. I suspect that, at a very subconscious level, it's one of the great drivers to look good.

Looking in the mirror involves looking at your own mortality. But it's also the reflection that you're most at home with. This reversed image is the one that's imprinted in your brain. It's why we feel more comfortable looking at our reflections than at photographs of ourselves.

When others look at you, they don't see you as you see yourself. They see a slightly different you—they see the photographic you. Which one is real? They both are.

CHAPTER FOUR

*Virtue! a fig! 'tis in ourselves that we are thus,
or thus. Our bodies are our gardens,
to the which our wills are gardeners.*

– *William Shakespeare,* Othello

BODY IMAGE

CAROLINE

Caroline tells a story that could have been penned by the Brothers Grimm. She saw herself as the goose in a family of swans. She grew up in a house with two very beautiful sisters. When she looked at them, she saw stunning, elegant faces set off with classic noses. She saw perfection.

When Caroline looked at herself, all she saw was a nose with a bump in it. She was personally sure it looked like a deformity. She obsessed about her nose, always looking for a hairstyle or blend of makeup that would divert attention from it. No one else remarked on it—not her parents, her friends, or her two sisters. But Caroline was convinced that they were just being nice.

When people talked about how beautiful "the sisters" were, she was sure they were talking about the beautiful sisters and including her out of politeness.

Caroline had a view of her appearance that appeared to be at odds with how others saw her.

ANNE

Anne is a tall, striking, 32-year-old woman with auburn hair, a quick wit, and a ready smile. The people who think she's beautiful include boys from high school ("I had my fair share of attention," she says), her husband, and her parents. She's always had a robust and enthusiastic cheering section.

So why, then, was Anne always trying to hide her face? When she stopped her car at a red light, she would look away so the complete stranger in the car beside her couldn't see her in profile. She had a problem with her nose. She believed it looked too much like her dad's nose—fine for him, but not for her.

Anne had one view of herself, while the people around her had another. Which one is real?

DISSATISFACTION WITH OURSELVES

You may be like Caroline and Anne. You're thinking about cosmetic surgery because you don't like something about your body. Perhaps, like Marie, your view of your body is shaped by how you see your parents. Marie, middle-aged and in good health, leads a very active life but felt that she was starting to look like her mother. It's not that she doesn't love her mother—she doesn't want to *become* her. It's a sign of mortality.

All women seem to have something they dislike about their bodies. In *Survival of the Prettiest*, Nancy Etcoff writes, "Every person knows the topography of her face and the landscape of her body as intimately as a mapmaker. To the outside world, we vary in small ways from our best hours to our worst. In our mind's eye, however, we undergo a kaleidoscope of changes and a bad hair day, a blemish or an added pound can undermine confidence in ways that equally minor fluctuations in our moods, our strength and our mental agility usually do not."

There is no such thing as a minor imperfection when it comes to the face or the body.

– Nancy Etcoff, psychologist

It's a major concern among women. It also turns out to be a large (and growing) concern among men. A 1972 survey by *Psychology Today* revealed that 23 percent of women and 15 percent of men didn't like their overall appearances. By 1997, the level of dissatisfaction had risen to 56 percent of women and 43 percent of men. Our dissatisfaction with our appearances is on the rise—and the men are catching up, which I can verify from my growing number of male patients.

This dissatisfaction is part of normal, everyday angst. But there's a grey area that anyone considering cosmetic surgery should be aware of. If everything you do has to be exactly as planned, or you look in the mirror and see flaws undetectable by anyone else, or you're compulsive by nature, cosmetic surgery may not be for you.

Body Dysmorphic Disorder

The search for perfection can cross the line into an ailment called body dysmorphic disorder (BDD). Daniel McNeill, in his book *The Face: A Natural History*, refers to BDD as "delusions of ugliness," best exemplified in Pablo Picasso's painting *Girl Before a Mirror*. A young blonde woman stares into the looking glass at a grotesque caricature. Her reflection is darker, her forehead blotched, and her hair green. "She's gazing at a chimera," McNeill says. "Her mind has warped her face."

In my experience, BDD can affect people to varying degrees, and among those who become obsessed with an imagined defect, no amount of plastic surgery can help. I've encountered patients who are absolutely certain that they have a terrible deformity of the nose when no such deformity exists. Medical literature is filled with cases of BDD. When invited to draw self-portraits, BDD sufferers invariably produce cartoonish depictions of their perceived deformities.

McNeill reports on one woman who hated her hair even though friends asked her for her stylist's name, hoping to duplicate it. Such unfortunate people's self-image problems lie elsewhere. Some research suggests that it's psychological and that many people with BDD were teased about their looks as children. People with BDD are frequently diagnosed with real depression, the kind that's often treated with drugs and therapy. In such cases, no amount of cosmetic surgery will help. I always tell prospective patients who appear to be depressed that cosmetic surgery isn't for them—at least, not right now.

Self-Image

In one scientific study of self-image, subjects were asked to grade their own images and those of friends in two ways: first in the mirror, and second in a photograph. The findings: We like our own images better when we view them in a mirror while our friends prefer photographs of us. Why is that? It's simply because we're drawn to the images that are most familiar to us. You're most comfortable looking at the reversed, reflected image of you. Others see you differently.

Paul Valéry believed we all have a three-body problem:

– First is the body we possess and inhabit—the self that we experience.
– Second is the body we present to the world—the one we dress and decorate.
– Third is our interior physical machine—the one we never see.

THE PSYCHOLOGICAL EFFECTS OF PLASTIC SURGERY

John and Marcia Goin, a surgeon-psychiatrist team who have studied the psychological effects of plastic surgery, say beauty isn't in the eye of the beholder but in the mind of the beheld. What do they mean?

Every face is unique, but all people seeking cosmetic surgery seem to have one thing in common. They feel they're somehow outside the normal range of where they want to be. They don't want to be more beautiful than their next-door neighbors or appear in *Vogue* magazine. Blending in means moving from a group they consider unacceptable ("not them") to a group that's acceptable. It's a subtle but profound concept.

On the surface it seems inconsistent, but it actually makes sense. If you feel as though you're in a group to which you don't belong and want to move into another more acceptable group, that shift carries with it the need for secrecy.

Here's the logic: If everyone knows you've joined the new, acceptable group because of surgery, you'll feel that you've made your way there under false pretenses. That shouldn't be the case, but it is.

I see evidence of this all the time. Patients feel better about themselves after they've dealt with something they don't like about their appearance. They're happier and more animated, and they project that in their behavior. Others respond, not to the work they've had done, but to that change in behavior. They're not reacting to the reshaped nose; they're reacting to the patient's reaction to the reshaped nose.

On the day of her surgery, Anne may have felt that she was jumping off a cliff, but now she feels like part of the group. It's as if her features are finally as they were meant to be. It usually takes two or three months for this to happen.

Some people don't like a particular feature, such as a bump on the nose or a bulbous tip. When we improve the things they don't like, then—in their mind's eye—this is the way they've always wanted to be and the way that they feel they are. Some psychologists would say that it's bizarre, that this shouldn't be, that what you are is what you are. Others would say you should be happy with your appearance because it's what God gave you.

But the reality is that people think of themselves with their nicer noses as looking the way they were meant to look. This *is* the real them. And they get into that new feeling very quickly.

Caroline had rhinoplasty and called it the best decision she could have made. "I no longer feel like the girl behind the huge nose," she says. "When people comment on how beautiful my sisters and I are, I actually believe that I'm really included in that. I feel 100 percent better about myself."

Caroline didn't just wake up one morning and decide to undergo rhinoplasty. As we've seen, the decision-making process is more complicated than that. But the final decision to go ahead is often triggered by something no more significant than a stranger's glance.

CHAPTER FIVE

Some younger cousins referred to my nose as looking like a witch's nose. I thought, "That's it! I'm getting this surgery ASAP."

— **Brad,** rhinoplasty and chin-implant patient

THE TURNING POINT

INDECISION AND DELAY

Perhaps you look older than you feel. Perhaps something about your facial features has bothered you for years. Either way, you've decided that cosmetic surgery may be for you.

You've progressed slowly through the early steps. You no longer dismiss the idea as outlandish. You're thinking about it. In fact, you've done some research and have even been in touch with people who have had face-lifts or rhinoplasty. The feedback is positive. You've even raised the subject, however tentatively, with your nearest and dearest, and the roof hasn't fallen in.

But something is still holding you back. That's understandable. Nobody rushes into a face-lift or rhinoplasty. You're not sure what it is you're waiting for, but you wait.

"I always hated my nose," Anne says. "Fixing it was something I wanted to do badly since I was a teenager. But I was always afraid of ending up with a little pinched Barbie nose." Anne waited and worried and waited some more. She finally had rhinoplasty at the age of thirty. It had taken her fourteen years to "jump off the cliff."

Mary first thought about having her eyes done in her thirties but always talked herself out of it. "I kept thinking I was being really selfish and superficial," she says. "I told myself it wasn't my looks but my character and my personality that were important." It took Mary twenty years, and by then she was ready, not just for work on her eyes, but for a face-lift.

Doreen booked her face-lift a full year in advance, but as the surgery date approached, she canceled. Then she did the same thing again. "I canceled twice and then was sorry afterwards," she says. "I just couldn't make that final step—but eventually, I did."

There's always a reason not to have cosmetic surgery, even for those who have been thinking seriously about it and researching it for many years. Rhinoplasty and other contour-altering procedures are usually performed on younger patients, predominantly women. Anne was thirty when she had her rhinoplasty. Facial rejuvenation surgery usually comes a few decades later, when patients are in their mid- to late forties and older. Mary was fifty-eight when she had her face-lift.

Sylvia wasn't forty-five or even fifty-five when she had her face-lift. She was seventy before she finally went ahead.

"My responsibility was always to my husband and children," she says. "I finally decided that this was something I could do just for me."

Differences between Men and Women

The long delay in coming to a decision, often fueled by guilt, is common, especially in women. They're the nurturers, the care-givers. Their focus is most often directed outward toward loved ones. As Kimberly puts it, "When you're in your life and raising children, you're not thinking about yourself." It often seems as if there's no room in that life for yourself. You have to make room, and that takes courage.

Men, on the other hand, are much more matter-of-fact. They decide on a course of action, forge ahead, get it done, and move on to other things. Men may have facial rejuvenation sur-gery because their wives did it, or they saw something on televi-sion, or somebody made a "you're looking old" remark. They might have puffy eyes and say to themselves, "I'll do this because there's a big downsizing coming in the company. I look old. I bet-ter do something about this."

Dave is a case in point. He's in his early fifties, and his wife Angie is just a few years younger. It isn't a May-December pair-ing, but you wouldn't know that from looking at them. With her Mediterranean features, smooth olive skin, and lustrous black hair, Angie wears her years well. Dave suffers from what you might call the "Curse of the Northern European." The dashing, fair-haired, and pale-skinned youth of three decades ago, the one who turned young women's heads, seems to have aged before his time. His blond locks have whitened and thinned, his chiseled features have sagged, and his fair skin has wrinkled and red-dened. Dave looks ten years older than he is.

Men usually don't go through the same process as women. They come in, ask about it, make a decision, go ahead and do it—and forget about it three weeks later. It's sometimes difficult to get them back for their follow-up appointments.

In their book *Why Men Don't Listen and Women Can't Read Maps*, internationally regarded business consultants Barbara and Allan Pease say that it comes down to male and female awareness. Male awareness is concerned with "getting results, achieving goals, status and power, beating the competition and getting efficiently to the bottom line." Female awareness is focused on "communication, co-operation, harmony, love, sharing and our relationship to one another."

THE TRIGGER EVENT

It's no wonder that people stew about face-lifts. The idea of doing something just for themselves is often far outside their normal range of experience. It takes a jolt—a pivotal event—to jump-start them into action. The turning point or trigger event can be a life-changing moment or a stranger's offhand remark.

Dave was dragged into a boutique by his wife. "When a saleslady told me that I had a gorgeous daughter, she didn't real-ize that she was talking about my wife," he recalls. "That was the last straw." That remark tipped him over the edge. He was ready to take action.

The turning point can occur unexpectedly during the most commonplace event. Anita always looked young for her age. She was one of those fresh-faced young women who look like teenagers all through their twenties. By her early fifties, Anita still looked much younger. She considered cosmetic surgery but always put it off. One morning, Anita took a mirror off the wall to clean behind it. She placed the mirror on a table—and looked down. "My whole face was sagging," she says. "I knew I had to do something about it."

For Doreen, it was a routine trip to the security office at work for a new photo identification card. She took one look at the picture that rolled out of the machine and decided to go ahead with her long-planned and twice-canceled face-lift.

One trigger event I encounter often is "The Shocking Revelation of the Wedding." You're a guest at someone's wedding, dressed to the nines, and having a fabulous time. At the reception, a wedding photographer is on the prowl. But that's okay. He has no interest in you. His focus is on the happy couple. Weeks later, you see the results: beautiful photos of a beautiful bride . . . and in three or four pictures, in the crowd, you at your worst. The camera has been kind to the bride and cruel to you. Where did those jowls come from? And what about those sagging eyes? It must be the light! But you realize it isn't the light. You look at the last picture and decide then and there, "That's it." You've reached your turning point.

That's what happened to Christina, who went to a co-worker's wedding. The pictures were passed around the office. "As I stared at the pictures in front of me, all I could manage to concentrate on was how terrible my nose looked and how it didn't seem to fit in with the rest of my facial features." Christina went back to her desk, sat down, and realized for the first time that she didn't have to live with her nose this way forever. That was her turning point.

Arpi has two daughters. "My eureka moment was at my older daughter's wedding. I was looking at the pictures, not the frontal shots but the profiles, and I thought, 'Good grief, that's a big honker.'" She resolved to put matters right before her younger daughter's wedding.

For some, that moment comes at a landmark birthday. Natasha decided on her fiftieth birthday. For Jean, it followed dental work. It seemed perfectly acceptable to have her teeth straightened. Why not her nose?

For many, more serious events will trigger the decision to go ahead. For Kimberly, it was her ordeal with breast cancer. "The cancer pushed me to do it," she says of the surgery she had at age fifty-six to correct a crooked nose. "When I recovered and I knew everything was going to be all right, I thought, 'Okay, now I'll do this. I'm living, thank goodness.'"

Adds Kim, "I decided to spend money on something that's not necessary for my physical health, though I think it *was* necessary for my mental health. I think my life would have been a lot better if I'd done it in my twenties. It would have given me more confidence."

Matthew decided after learning he had prostate cancer. "I really started to reflect on my life, on the fact that life is truly short and that we all should do what we want to, live life to the fullest, and hope not to have many regrets for not having done things."

Sylvia says she'd been toying with the idea of cosmetic surgery for years. She decided on September 11, 2001. "We watched it all on TV, and I said to my husband, 'I'm not going to wait. I'm going to do it now.'"

Sylvia wasn't alone. It may seem odd or out of place, but many people made the same decision on that terrible day.

You've moved from thinking about cosmetic surgery and researching it. You've had your "eureka moment," and have decided to take action. What now? The next big step is finding the right doctor.

CHAPTER SIX

Success depends upon previous preparation,
and without such preparation
there is sure to be failure.

— *Confucius*, philosopher

FINDING THE RIGHT DOCTOR

You've come a long way—from dismissing the idea of cosmetic surgery as a pipe dream . . . to thinking about it as something that you could do . . . to telling someone close to you that you're considering it . . . to making the decision to go ahead. Even at this stage, it's been a long journey, full of misgivings, second thoughts, and angst.

Now you have to find a doctor—not just any doctor, but an experienced doctor who specializes in the kind of surgery you're going to have. Beyond that, your chosen doctor must inspire your confidence. You have to be able to tell yourself, "I can trust this doctor with my face."

You often ask yourself: Which doctor is right for me? How will I know? How many doctors should I see before deciding on one? It seems like a daunting task, but it's quite manageable. With a little detective work, you'll soon find yourself face-to-face with the doctor who is right for you.

DOING YOUR RESEARCH

Start by asking around. Word of mouth is one of the best ways to determine which doctors should be on your short list. A third of the people who come through my door have heard about me from my patients.

You probably have a friend, relative, or co-worker who has had plastic surgery and won't mind talking about it. Find out if he or she is satisfied with the results. Start a list of trusted doctors. You'll be surprised at how quickly you get names. Andrea approached a trusted work colleague who had had rhinoplasty and took it from there.

Talk to your family doctor. He or she will almost certainly know of several cosmetic surgeons. Add them to your list. Nurses are also a good source of information. Marie spoke to a nurse who knew the buzz about cosmetic surgeons and provided her with a short list of favorites. Determine which names keep appearing. Check with your local medical association. They'll have a list of approved and certified facial plastic surgeons. Compare that list with the one you've been making. By now you should have a list of several facial plastic surgeons whose names keep coming up.

Take your sleuthing a step further. Go on the Internet, review web pages, and browse chat rooms (but be careful here, as they aren't always accurate). See who's being quoted in newspaper and magazine articles. Milla started her list from a lifestyle magazine article listing the top ten cosmetic surgeons in her city. Sarah asked her aesthetician, as she believed that they (along with hairdressers) know a thing or two about who are the "in" surgeons in town.

Price, although important, wasn't the deciding factor. Qualifications, professionalism, and personality were. After all, this was my face.

– *Katherine,* face-lift patient

CHECKING CREDENTIALS

By now you should have a list of names. But you're not yet ready to decide. This is your raw data. You're now ready to do your due diligence by checking the medical credentials of the top two or three names on your list. This process has two key steps:

- Make sure that your doctor is certified in his or her specialty.
- Determine if he or she specializes in the procedures that you're interested in.

At first glance, it may seem like a difficult and confusing task. You'll discover any or all of the following:

- Plastic surgeons who operate everywhere on the body, including face-lifts, breast implants, tummy tucks, liposuction, and a lot more

- Facial plastic surgeons who specialize in facial work
- Ophthalmologists who do oculoplastic surgery (plastic surgery around the eye)
- Otolaryngologists who have specific training in head and neck surgery
- Dermatologists who do reconstructive work on patients recovering from cancer surgery, as well as other cosmetic treatments (e.g., facial fillers, Botox, lasers)
- Oral surgeons who specialize in upper and lower jaw surgery to improve facial deformities, which can be both cosmetic and reconstructive
- A host of specialties, subspecialties, and superspecialties
- An alphabet soup of initials after doctors' names

Several different types of specialists provide excellent cosmetic surgery care. All have completed medical school (or dental school, for oral surgeons) and some type of specialty training (surgical or medical). Many will have taken superspecialty training in cosmetic surgery. Most surgeons train for twelve to seventeen years, which involves at least eighty hours a week.

Consider Joan Smith, a fictional plastic surgeon whose education and training is typical for doctors in this field. Joan graduates from university with an undergraduate degree in science. She's accepted to medical school. She spends four years learning about anatomy, physiology, and pathology in various body organs. As Joan progresses through medical school, she does increasing amounts of clinical work—seeing patients in the hospital—under the watchful eye of physician teachers. By her fourth year, she's doing a clinical clerkship, working as a junior member on a team with her work being overseen.

Joan gets a medical degree but isn't ready to see patients on her own yet. She must decide if she wants to go into general practice or pursue a medical or surgical specialty. For general practice in family medicine, she would go into a two- or three-year residency and pass exams before being certified as a family doctor.

But Joan wants to go into facial plastic surgery. Specialty training takes four to seven years. Joan chooses the specialty of otolaryngology—head and neck surgery that includes facial plastic surgery. Joan's training lasts at least eleven or twelve years—three or four undergraduate years, plus four years at medical school, plus four or more specialist years. As part of her superspecialty training, Joan writes several certification exams and may do a fellowship with a practising facial plastic surgeon. She'll be at least thirty years old before she's ready to begin independent practice.

Medical Boards and Associations

If you have any doubt or concern about the credentials of a doctor on your short list, check with the professional associations that represent plastic surgeons. There are many different certifying or credentialing boards and colleges, regulatory and licensing boards, academies, and associations. The list below contains information on some of the associations you should know about.

American Academy of Facial Plastic and Reconstructive Surgery (AAFPRS)

- The world's largest professional association of facial plastic and reconstructive surgeons. Most members have their specialty in otolaryngology—head and neck surgery, and some specialize in facial plastic surgery.

- Provides continuing medical education courses, represents the specific interests of its members to the public, and educates the public about the work of its specialists in facial plastic surgery.
- Many Canadian surgeons are also members of this academy.
- Can provide a list of surgeons by region who are board-certified to perform facial plastic and reconstructive surgery.
- Call 1-800-332-FACE or visit www.facemd.org for more information.

American Board of Facial Plastic and Reconstructive Surgery (ABFPRS)
- The certifying board for facial plastic surgeons in the U.S. and Canada.
- Visit www.abfprs.org for more information.

American Board of Medical Specialities (ABMS)
- An umbrella organization that assists twenty-four medical specialty boards in the development and use of standards.It is the largest entity overseeing physician certification in the United States.
- Call 1-866-275-2267 or visit www.abms.org to confirm a doctor's certification in a recognized medical specialty.
- Note: Some highly credible specialty boards, such as the ABFPRS, are not members of the ABMS.

American Medical Association (AMA) and Canadian Medical Association (CMA)
- Represent the majority of practising physicians and surgeons in the United States and Canada, respectively.

- These associations speak for the political and socioeconomic interests of their members and play a large part in educating the public about medicine.
- Visit www.ama-assn.org or www.cma.ca for more information.

American Society of Plastic and Reconstructive Surgery (ASPRS)
- Equivalent American society to the AAFPRS for plastic surgeons who do body cosmetic surgery as well as facial surgery.
- Visit www.plasticsurgery.org for more information.

Canadian Academy of Facial Plastic and Reconstructive Surgery (CAFPRS)
- The Canadian equivalent to the AAFPRS for facial plastic surgeons.
- Visit www.facialcosmeticsurgery.org for more information.

Canadian Society of Aesthetic Plastic Surgery
- Canadian society for Plastic Surgeons who do body and facial cosmetic sugery.
- Visit www.csaps.ca for more information.

Federation of State Medical Boards (FSMB)
- In the U.S., the FSMB keeps track of the status of doctors' medical licences and maintains records of disciplinary actions against doctors.
- To check a doctor's credentials, call 1-817-868-4000 or visit www.fsmb.org.

Royal College of Physicians and Surgeons (RCPS)
- The certifying body for medical and surgical specialists in Canada.

– To qualify as a fellow of the RCPS, candidates must pass a credentialing examination.

– Call 1-800-668-3740 or visit rcpsc.medical.org for more information.

State Medical Boards and Provincial Colleges

– These are the state or provincial licensing boards for physicians and surgeons.

– Check your state or province for contact information.

Certification

The ABFPRS is the certifying board for facial plastic surgery. Both American and Canadian otolaryngologists—head and neck surgeons and plastic surgeons are eligible. Other surgeons certified by their otolaryngology—head and neck surgery or plastic surgery boards may also specialize in facial plastic surgery. To be certified by these organizations, doctors must have gone through extensive plastic and reconstructive surgery training and residency, and passed comprehensive written and oral examinations. Some ophthalmologists specialize in oculoplastic or ophthalmic plastic surgery around the eye. They're certified by the ABMS in the United States and RCPS in Canada.

In the United States, a physician or surgeon can usually receive a state medical licence to practice in his or her specialty once his or her residency training is completed. In Canada, a surgeon must complete the training program and pass a credentialing exam through the RCPS to obtain his or her FRCSC (Fellow of the Royal College of Surgeons of Canada). A doctor who is board-certified by the ABFPRS in the United States or

Canada is a specialist in facial plastic surgery. In the United States, the doctor will, as a prerequisite, be certified by the ABMS in otolaryngology—head and neck surgery or plastic surgery. In Canada, the doctor will also require primary certification by the RCPS in either otolaryngology—head and neck surgery or plastic surgery.

The use of specialist titles is regulated to varying degrees in different states and provinces. "Cosmetic surgeons" may or may not have had formal plastic surgery training (or even surgical training).

SELECTING A DOCTOR

Selecting a physician from a given specialty is important. However, it's very important to select the physician or surgeon who has the most experience and best reputation for the particular treatments or surgery that you're seeking.

The most important factor should be your consultation with the doctor. Having a good rapport with your doctor will make you feel more at ease with the process. You should also feel confident that he or she can provide you with what you're seeking. If a particular physician has strong references and you're happy with him or her, it may not be necessary to visit two or three other doctors to compare. However, if you aren't comfortable or don't feel that your questions have been answered, make sure to see two or three other doctors before making your decision. This approach does have a downside. By seeing too many doctors, you may receive conflicting advice, which can sometimes make your decision-making process more difficult.

Red Flags

There are many excellent facial plastic surgeons. With a little care and research, you'll find the right one for you. However, plastic surgery has become a highly competitive business. Keep that in mind, and be wary of these warning signs:

- Extravagant promises: The goal should be improvement, not perfection. A doctor who promises perfection is promising too much and will almost certainly be unable to deliver.

- Advertising and bargain prices: Doctors can advertise their services and specialties, but be cautious about one who advertises extensively, especially if that doctor's fees are substantially lower than those of competitors. Good plastic surgeons don't have "specials." Beyond that, their new patients tend to come by way of patient or doctor referrals.

- The short consultation: The first visit with a plastic surgeon must be a thorough, get-to-know-you session in which both patient and doctor determine if they can work together. If you find yourself in a room viewing a video about the doctor's services and are whisked through a brief meeting, you may want to look elsewhere.

- Pressure tactics: A doctor should never pressure you to make a decision at an initial consultation.

- Prescribing unwanted treatment: If the doctor encourages you to have treatments or procedures you don't understand or don't feel you need, make your feelings known. Be prepared to walk away if it continues.

- Ignoring your interests: Some doctors may not put your best interests first. Your concerns should always take priority.

THE INITIAL CONSULTATION

How do you know if plastic surgery is right for you? How do I, as the doctor, know? The first meeting will help both the surgeon and patient to find the answer. Each will evaluate the other. The patient wonders, "Can I trust this doctor with my face?" The surgeon thinks, "Does the patient have the motivation and personality to go through with it successfully?"

By the end of the initial consultation, both parties should have their answers. If it isn't "yes" on both sides, proceed no further, or plan a second visit to review any concerns. As Victor Hugo said, "Caution is the elder child of wisdom." This journey is a partnership. You're going through it together. There has to be mutual trust. The patient must be aware of the risks and committed to following up. The doctor must know the patient's individual needs and feel confident that he or she can help.

I always begin by asking a patient to tell me about his or her face. It's a deliberately open-ended question, aimed at having the patient tell me what's bothering him or her. It's important that the patient, not the surgeon, identify the problem. The patient needs to say he or she is unhappy with the bags under his or her eyes, doesn't like the shape of his or her nose, and so on. The more specific the patient is, the better.

In our first meeting, I need to learn the following:
- How long the patient has been unhappy with the body part in question
- Why an operation is being considered now
- What the patient's motivations are for seeking out the surgery

- What the patient's expectations are about the effects on his or her life
- How family and friends feel about it
- What degree of support he or she has from family and friends
- If the patient is under any kind of stress
- What the patient's fears or concerns are

It seems like a lot, but the information is important if the doctor-patient partnership is to proceed successfully.

Marie was very specific at our first meeting. "My face is fine," she said. "I just want to look more rested." She went on to describe drooping in her eyelids, frown lines in her forehead, and a sagging neck. She talked about her busy lifestyle, which included running, cross-country skiing, weightlifting, Pilates, digital photography, reading and writing, and doing crossword puzzles.

Much of this may seem beside the point for a plastic surgeon. But it isn't. On an initial consultation, the surgeon wants to know what kind of life the patient is leading. Is the patient active, busy, and outgoing or quiet, sedate, and reflective? It isn't necessarily an if/then scenario (e.g., if he or she doesn't have an outgoing personality, then I won't do the surgery). But it does help in assessing whether a patient can go through with it and be happy with the results.

With her busy life, positive attitude, and realistic goals, Marie was a good candidate for cosmetic surgery and had a good result. But remember, she didn't just jump into it. She thought about it for a long time before moving ahead.

THE EVALUATION

A number of factors can help you to determine if you would be a good candidate for cosmetic surgery.

Motivation

If you aren't 100 percent clear on why you're doing it, you may want to stop and think about your reasons. Cosmetic facial surgery comes with no guarantee of love, prosperity, and happiness. If you're planning surgery to please someone else, put those plans on hold and rethink your motivation.

If you have a "contour problem," such as a nose that grew too big in adolescence, and you've only begun to dislike it in your thirties, you should ask yourself, "Why now and not before?" You may have other issues that rhinoplasty can't resolve.

If a patient says, "Doctor, I'm sort of unhappy with how I look. What can you do for me?" I take that as a warning sign. This person may not be ready for surgery or, more likely, may be struggling with some other problem. It's not the face—it's the marriage or something else. People considering cosmetic surgery must be clear about what it is about their faces that they find unsatisfactory. There are also the compulsive, the perfectionist, and the individual who's never satisfied. Such people are unlikely to be satisfied with cosmetic surgery, no matter how good the result. In some cases, this may be a sign of a psychological problem such as body dysmorphic disorder.

Depression

No amount of surgery will make a depressed person happy. If you suffer from clinical depression, which is more than the occasional bout of being down in the dumps, you shouldn't have cosmetic surgery. You'll still be depressed afterward. See your family doctor to deal with the depression, and then see how you feel about a face-lift.

Health

Cosmetic surgery isn't a do-or-die proposition. You don't have to have it to restore your health or save your life. As a result, the thorough preoperative health screening process will eliminate unsuitable candidates. For example, if you have hypertension or high blood pressure, you'll be advised to get it under control before proceeding with elective surgery. On the other hand, if you found yourself in the emergency room after a serious automobile accident and needed immediate surgery, that same hypertension would be well within the bounds of acceptable risk.

Some people, such as hemophiliacs, aren't good candidates for elective surgery. Others can become candidates with some preparation, including the following:

- Smokers: Most of my patients have given up smoking. Not smoking, following a healthy diet, and getting plenty of exercise are all part of their lifestyles—and plastic surgery is part of that continuum. For those who still smoke, you need to stop at least two weeks before surgery. Smokers take longer to heal and undergo greater risk during surgery.
- The overweight: You may need to shed some pounds. But here's the upside. You can make a diet and exercise regimen part of your new healthy lifestyle—all of it enhanced by the surgery you'll have a few months down the line.

– The stressed: If you've just been laid off, fired, or divorced, plastic surgery may not be a good idea. This caution isn't limited to negative causes of stress. The good things in life bring their own kind of stress. If you've just married the love of your life, bought a house, or gotten a big promotion, you may also want to let things settle down before moving ahead with plastic surgery.

If, after thorough deliberation, you find you're truly ready for change, what next? Are you ready for surgery? You might first consider some non-surgical procedures, also known as minimally or non-invasive treatments.

CHAPTER SEVEN

*Beauty, to me, is about being comfortable
in your own skin.
That, or a kick-ass red lipstick.*

— *Gwyneth Paltrow,* actress

SKIN CARE FROM SUNBLOCK TO SANDBLASTING

You're at lunch with a friend. You excuse yourself and slip into the washroom. There, you witness a bewildering sight: a woman making faces at herself in the mirror. She alternately raises her brows and frowns. The movements are elaborate and exaggerated: a look of startled surprise followed by the world's biggest frown, repeated over and over.

Is she in the grip of some neurological disorder? Has she taken leave of her senses? Should you flee? The answers are no, no, and no. You're witnessing a Botox moment.

The woman has just had—probably within the last thirty minutes—perhaps half a dozen Botox injections in her upper face. The mugging at the mirror is a post-injection routine to help ensure that it settles in the right place and does its job of weakening the muscles that causes frown lines between the eyes.

Botox is one of several nonsurgical ways to diminish lines in the face and improve sagging in certain areas. The others include temporary fillers, such as Juvéderm^{TM}**, Restylane®†, or one of the other dozens of fillers on the market. Every doctor has his or her preferred filler. These products are used for aging skin to smoothen wrinkles, soften furrows, and add volume to deflated tissues.

COMMON SENSE TIPS

- Don't smoke. Aside from the damage it causes to the heart and lungs, smoking ages and wrinkles skin.
- Always use sunblock with SPF (sun protection factor) 30 or higher. SPF measures the amount of sun protection provided by sunblock. SPF 30 means that you can spend thirty times as much time in the sun to get the same exposure as you would without sunblock.
- Wear a hat. If you're a forty-year-old with a tan, you may look great now, but the damage from all that sun exposure will come back to haunt you. By the time you're fifty-five, you'll look much older. Beyond that, getting skin cancer is also a very real danger.

MAINTAINING THE SKIN

You can do plenty of things to maintain your skin quality before you need to turn to fillers and Botox. Let's start with the simplest, least invasive options. Some of these are known as "lunchtime" procedures. You can have them done and go right back to work.

Exfoliants and Moisturizers

Study the skin on your face in the mirror. The skin you see wasn't there six months ago. Cells grow in the lower layer of the skin, move up to the outer layer, die, flake off, and are replaced by new skin cells. This process of regeneration goes on constantly.

The easiest way to take care of your skin involves creams that exfoliate the skin's surface, such as vitamin A or glycolic acid creams. All you're doing is taking off dead cells. It's neither dramatic nor permanent, but it produces a nice look.

You can also use moisturizers, which work in one of two ways: They're either hydrophobic or hydrophilic (*hydro* means "water," *phobic* means "fear," and *philic* means "love"). Hydrophobic moisturizers create a barrier that prevents water from evaporating from the skin, while hydrophilic moisturizers attract water to the skin. Both plump up the skin and help to prevent very fine wrinkles from showing. The results won't be dramatic, but they'll help the skin to appear softer and more hydrated.

I will buy any creme, cosmetic, or elixir from a woman with a European accent.

– Erma Bombeck, humorist

Skin Peels

Visit an aesthetician for a glycolic acid peel. This will provide a deeper level of exfoliation. The skin peel feels a little tingly when it goes on and leaves your face with a rosy or pinkish hue.

A glycolic acid peel is a good option when you don't want downtime—you're busy enough as it is! Sometimes television programs exaggerate the truth to create humor. For example, one episode of *Sex and the City* shows Samantha joining her friends for lunch and stating that she has just had a peel done. Her face looks very red and raw, much to the horror of her friends. This isn't accurate! After a typical chemical peel, the pink hue will quickly dissipate. With a stronger peel, some people may experience slight flaking after a few days—which is easily helped with the application of moisturizer—but that's it. What you're left with is glowing, fresh skin.

Store-bought skin peels are usually buffered and available in an 8 to 10 percent concentration. Aestheticians may use a glycolic acid peel with a concentration of 30 to 50 percent. If used within a doctor's office, they can go as high as 70 percent concentration. Higher concentration means higher strength.

Microdermabrasion

Microdermabrasion works like a miniature sandblaster: It blows aluminum oxide crystals onto the skin and vacuums them up. The process removes old skin cells and stimulates production of collagen, the skin's structural protein. Microdermabrasion is often used in combination with skin peels. They're usually provided over three to five treatments, two to three weeks apart. Microdermabrasion smoothes fine wrinkles, improves superficial skin pigmentation, and gives the skin a healthier glow.

The bottom-line benefit of having either microdermabrasion or a skin peel is that they both help to reveal more glowing, radiant skin with minimal or no downtime.

IPL Photorejuvenation

IPL (intense pulsed light) photorejuvenation can reduce brown spots caused by sun exposure or red blotches from small broken blood vessels in the face. It's very effective for improving the skin on areas other than the face, such as the cleavage and the backs of the hands. It works on small facial skin imperfections. IPL photorejuvenation is also a treatment for rosacea, a common skin ailment that leaves people red-faced from dilated blood vessels and flushing.

The process begins with you lying down, wearing dark glasses to protect your eyes from the bright light. A cold gel is applied to the area to be treated. The handheld IPL glass surface is placed on the skin, and then pulses of light are applied. You might feel a slight sting. The entire procedure takes about twenty minutes. You may need several treatments, with a regular maintenance treatment every three to six months. After the first treatment, your skin might peel slightly.

Most women love the result of having more even skin tone. It reduces the need for using foundation to help create the often-desired "flawless" complexion.

THE LASER

The laser is the closest thing to the fountain of youth. It makes the skin more youthful. Even under a microscope, lasered skin can appear up to fifteen years younger.

A carbon dioxide (CO_2) laser, applied to the face, produces pulses of light that vaporize the skin one layer at a time. The skin is gently wiped away to reveal the layer beneath. The laser resurfaces the skin by stimulating collagen. It makes it possible to change the facial tissue without making an incision. As a result, the laser can

- resurface the skin, regardless of age
- remove some wrinkles, especially around the mouth and eyes
- remove age spots, superficial skin cancers, and other irregularities on sun-damaged skin
- improve scarring from acne, accidents, or previous surgery
- remove benign facial lesions

After laser treatment, the collagen in the skin will keep regenerating for up to eighteen months. As a result, the skin actually becomes more youthful. Under a microscope, the skin of a fifty-year-old who's had laser treatment can look like the skin of a thirty-five-year-old. It's a very powerful tool.

This is no lunchtime procedure. You must prepare your skin up to two weeks ahead of the procedure with exfoliants and demelanizing agents. This involves applying a retinoic acid cream that produces a mild facial peel (e.g., Retin A), a mild skin bleach (e.g., hydroquinone), and a steroid cream (e.g., hydrocortisone). You must also take an antiviral drug (e.g., Valtrex) and an antibiotic (e.g., cloxacillin) ahead of time.

The procedure is usually done under anesthetic. During recovery, you'll have to keep your head elevated as much as possible and apply Polysporin, Vaseline, or some other topical chosen by your doctor to improve healing. You'll also have to keep a low profile. Your face may be swollen and crusty for about a week. This will subside, and then you'll look salmon-pink for several weeks. This can be masked with camouflage makeup. When healing is complete, you'll look younger. Healing time can be shortened by reducing the energy in the laser, but there's a trade-off: The results aren't as good.

Other Laser Options

There are now a range of options for laser resurfacing:

- Non-ablative lasers (e.g., Smoothbeam): They don't vaporize the surface of the skin but still stimulate collagen production. They leave the epidermis (the outer layer of skin) intact.
- Fractional lasers (e.g., SmartXide®): They vaporize tiny sections of skin, leaving adjacent areas untouched. This "checkerboarding" approach speeds up healing because normal undamaged skin is interspersed with treated areas.
- Combination lasers (e.g., Fraxel® Re:store): They're both non-ablative (they don't vaporize the surface of the skin) and fractional (they stimulate the collagen underneath).

These lasers have faster healing times and fewer potential complications than CO_2 lasers, but the results aren't as good. The CO_2 laser is still the gold standard for skin resurfacing. However, the trend is toward fractional laser resurfacing because many patients are willing to accept a lesser result for less downtime and less risk of complications. Innovative research and new technologies hold the promise of even better laser options in the years to come.

Each wrinkle is unique.
They're like orgasms. Some are deep.
Some are shallow. Others make you scream.

— *Joan Rivers*, comedian

FILLERS

Fillers are injections that restore volume to the curves of the face and smooth out wrinkles. They're becoming more and more popular. Some people call them the "liquid face-lift" because they can take years off an aging face for much less than the cost of surgery.

Temporary fillers (such as Juvéderm and Restylane) are made from hyaluronic acid (HA), a substance found naturally in the skin. Typically fillers last from nine to twelve months. HA fillers (or HAs) come in different grades or viscosities that range from thinner to thicker:

- Thinner (finer) grades are used for the most superficial wrinkles, such as crow's feet, "smoker's lines" in the lips, and fine cheek or forehead creases.
- Medium grades are used for cheek-lip furrows caused by a sagging cheek, cheek-mouth lines (sometimes called "sad" or "marionette" lines), and other moderate facial furrows.
- Thicker (heavier) grades are used for very deep furrows or for volume filling. With aging, the facial skin droops due to loss of elastic tone and gravity. It also loses volume (which is known as "deflation"). You can see this in the loss of cheek prominence, the hollow under the eyes (called a "tear trough"), and in the depression in front of the jaw. These

areas can often be dramatically improved by injecting higher volumes of filler to replace the natural loss of tissue volume. Excellent long-term results can be achieved, with most patients maintaining these corrections for one to two years (or more).

Many people worry about the pain or discomfort associated with these types of injections. There are several ways to decrease pain or discomfort, such as using cool compresses, topical anesthetic, vibrating instruments, and squeezable "stress balls." Some fillers contain a local anesthetic, or patients may have local anesthetic injected first. Most people rate the pain or discomfort from being injected with a temporary filler as a 2 to 4 out of 10 (with 10 being the worst pain).

Permanent fillers are becoming less popular. Though some have been relatively effective, the newer temporary fillers are lasting longer, providing improved aesthetic results. Most plastic surgeons and dermatologists are coming to favor temporary fillers over permanent fillers, as they have a lower risk of complications.

Fillers are an increasingly popular way to change your appearance without surgery, and many types are in use. Besides HA, fillers are made from animal collagen, calcium, and synthetics. These various types all work. Examples include the following:

– Radiesse™: This filler works on laugh lines and other facial wrinkles, and can also be used to change the shape of the chin, nose, and cheeks. It's made from a calcium compound found naturally in bones and teeth. Dentists and orthopedic surgeons have been using versions of this filler for many years.

– Sculptra: This synthetic filler treats the deep folds between the nose and mouth, folds around the corners of the mouth, sunken cheeks, wrinkles in the cheeks or chin, and even deep scars. It's made from a chemical that's been in use for years in dissolving surgical sutures.

As with all fillers, the challenge is to place the right amount smoothly in the correct skin layer to achieve a natural look. With most cosmetic medical treatments, the product is only part of what determines the final result. It's important to seek out a physician with the experience and "artistic" skill to ensure that your results look natural and simply enhance your beauty.

BOTOX

Botox is the nonsurgical cosmetic treatment that everyone talks about. It's the stock-in-trade of television entertainment shows and late-night comedians. Who's had work? Is it the Botox or is it just Cher? One of my patients is an entertainment lawyer who spends a lot of time in Los Angeles. "I've never seen so many beautiful, frozen faces," she tells me. Another patient says Botox produces a too-smooth forehead that she calls "the bald look."

I suspect the name alone has much to do with people's skittish reactions. Botox! There's something scary about it—more so when you stretch it out to its full, slightly menacing length: botulinum toxin. It evokes plague-like images of bad summer disaster movies in which people run for their lives and Bruce Willis wears a hazmat suit. But, injected in the right places and in the right amounts, Botox works.

Again, it's important to reiterate that you're wise to seek out an experienced, skilled physician to ensure that you get the best, most natural-looking results. Botox requires a physician who has a solid knowledge of facial anatomy, the gift of an "aesthetic eye" for each patient, and years of experience to ultimately create a "fresh" and "relaxed" look. When a skilled, experienced physician treats you with Botox, you look like yourself . . . at your best!

Proven History of Botox Medical Use

The reality of Botox is that it's been in safe use for more than twenty years. Injected, it will temporarily relax or paralyze specific muscles under the skin, making it useful for many non-cosmetic procedures and the treatment of various medical conditions. People with painful ailments such as cervical dystonia (involuntary contractions or spasms of the neck muscles) can get relief from a Botox injection. The same goes for blepharospasm (the involuntary blinking caused by spasms of the muscles controlling the eyelid) or strabismus (a cross-eyed condition in which one eye turns inward). Health Canada has approved the use of Botox in treating cerebral palsy in children as young as two years old. The medical uses go on and on. Botox relieves a lot of suffering. Several of my patients report that it helps with their migraines.

The amount of Botox used for cosmetic applications is significantly less than the amounts used to therapeutically treat medical conditions. In fact, most medical treatments use many times the amount of Botox used in cosmetic treatments. This only emphasizes how safe Botox is for cosmetic use. Long-term safety data are published and available for anyone interested in learning more about Botox. The future will likely see other types of botulium toxin developed.

Cosmetic Applications

Many patients tell me the same thing: "I'm constantly being told by my family and friends that I look tired or stressed . . . but honestly, I feel just fine! I don't like what I see in the mirror, as it doesn't reflect how I feel inside." Sometimes, expression lines convey emotions that others will interpret as anger, worry, or stress—even when you don't feel any of these. Many muscles contribute to expression.

In cosmetic use, Botox works best in areas where muscles are dynamic. ("Dynamic" refers to the action where muscles contract and move under the skin, which causes the skin to fold and wrinkle.) Some of the most dynamic lines are located between the eyebrows above the nose (also known as the *glabella*). Botox is most commonly used here to raise a droopy eyebrow or smooth out forehead wrinkles and furrows. It's also very effective in diminishing the crow's feet caused by squinting and "bunny lines" caused by turning up the nose. It can decrease a "gummy smile," create fuller lips, and decrease "smoker's lines" around the mouth. Botox helps to raise the droopy corners of the mouth and can eliminate the dimply *peau d'orange* (or "orange skin") look in the chin. It can decrease jowling in some people to improve the jaw line (the "Nefertiti Lift"), decrease neck muscle banding, and decrease the square-jawed look of those with hyperactive or large chewing muscles.

More uses for Botox are being discovered every year. More than 3,000 studies of Botox have been done over the last ten years (more than any other drug) to ensure its efficacy and long-term safety. If Botox-related problems occur, it's usually for one of two reasons:

– Inexperienced doctors who don't know how to administer it

– Over-aggressive doctors who administer too much

You can use Botox to reduce a muscle's action or completely relax that muscle for three to four months. Botox is used in very small amounts in specific muscles to achieve a natural, fresh look.

For example, the glabella (the smooth part of the forehead above the line of the eyebrows) is one of the most expressive parts of the face. Those expressions can turn into "angry lines" with age. Botox injections can diminish the lines for three months or longer; a lot of Botox can smooth those lines out. Others will stop asking, "What's the matter?", "What are you worried about?" or "Why are you angry?" Recent studies have shown that patients not only look less worried but also actually feel better.

Botox amounts are measured in units. I will frequently give six injections in the forehead, each one containing a minimum of 2.5 units of Botox. That's a total of 15 units. It's often enough to relax the muscle without creating a frozen look, but many patients require more. Many patients receive at least 20 units (and sometimes 30 or 40 units) in the glabella. You want to have enough to create the "look" the patient wants.

My philosophy isn't to use as much Botox as I can or to use so much that the muscle doesn't move at all. I believe the goal should be to make a person look more relaxed and youthful, and to use Botox to sculpt the action of the facial muscles. The aim is to create a natural and untreated look.

Today, it's also very common to use Botox and fillers together. Botox is used to diminish the activity of the dynamic muscles, while fillers are used to diminish wrinkles and furrows that are present even when the face is relaxed. Fillers complement treatment by replacing volume lost in the cheeks and other facial hollows. Fillers restore what nature has depleted over time. Studies show that the fillers last longer when combined with Botox therapy. Similarly, if laser therapy is being used to treat crow's feet or wrinkles around the mouth, the result will be better if Botox is first used to decrease the muscle action postoperatively.

BOTOX WEDNESDAY

Botox Wednesday is the day, usually twice a month, when patients come in for their injectibles (i.e., temporary fillers and Botox). It's a big day for everyone—including us because of what we learn from our patients. They'll report on what's working for them and what isn't. A patient getting Botox may not have quite the look he or she wants and we may slightly increase the amount this time around. The same goes for fillers.

On a typical Botox Wednesday . . .

– Jane is here for the fourth time. She's had injections in the forehead to diminish lines, but not entirely eliminate them. Now we move on, injecting a little Botox just above the outer part of the eyebrow. That minimizes the action of the depressor muscle, which means that the opposing muscle (the *frontalis*) gets a little more action. The effect is to ever-so-slightly increase the arch of the brow. She loves how it gives her eyes a more open, fresher look. She can now show off her eye makeup better.

- Mary-Anne, eighteen months after her face-lift, receives a series of Botox injections in the forehead, a little more on one side than on the other. My experienced aesthetic eye detects some natural asymmetry, which I attempt to address with the treatment. "It may not be perfect," I advise. "That's fine by me," she replies. "Perfect people don't need love. I do." At age fifty-one, Mary-Anne is going for the all-natural look—little or no makeup. "I can get away with it," she says. "People think I look ten years younger."

- Joanne, who's seventy years old, is troubled by the small lines along her upper lip. "I don't know why they give women drinks with straws in them," she says. She's injected with a small amount of the temporary filler Juvéderm.

As we've seen, you can do many things in conjunction with or instead of cosmetic facial surgery. Sometimes, as in Marguerite's case, you can do both at the same time. She had laser treatment on the lines around her mouth, along with a face-lift.

CHAPTER EIGHT

Dreams are renewable. No matter what our age or condition, there are still untapped possibilities within us and new beauty waiting to be born.

– *Dale Turner,* motivator

FACE-LIFTS

COMMON QUESTIONS ABOUT FACE-LIFTS

Surgery is a big deal, especially facial plastic surgery. It's one thing to go under the knife because you have a serious illness and no other options. It's another to voluntarily submit to a face-lift. You'll have many questions, and many of them should be answered below.

Will it hurt?

Most patients say that they feel little or no pain. But you'll feel miserable the morning after. Everything around your head will feel tender. It's not stung-by-a-hornet, rock-on-the-foot pain, but it's no walk in the park either. In fact, you won't feel like walking in the park for a few days. An over-the-counter medication that isn't aspirin-based (e.g., Tylenol) should suffice.

Doctors have a habit of substituting the word "discomfort" for "pain." For example, your doctor may say, "You're just going to feel a little discomfort." But one patient's discomfort is another patient's pain. That said, in most cases, there's very little actual pain. If you're "discomfortable" and need something stronger than Tylenol, prescription pain medication is available.

Will I feel sick?

You may be mildly nauseated from the anesthesia, which can take a day or two to leave your system. However, it's by no means a certainty. Not everyone experiences postoperative nausea. You may also feel weak, have occasional palpitations, get dizzy, and even break out in cold sweats. Beyond that, your temperature may be above normal (38.5 degrees Celsius or 100 degrees Fahrenheit). That's enough to make you a little feverish. Treat all of this with a lot of fluids (but no alcohol) and Tylenol (preferably extra-strength). The nausea, if present at all, will usually pass within a few hours.

Will I feel like crying?

You may feel a little down and anxious in the days after your surgery. Who wouldn't after what you've been through? You may switch on the TV and burst into tears during a commercial. You've received a shock to your body. Keep this in mind: You'll quickly get over it, and, every time you look in the mirror, you'll be glad you went through the surgery.

What about swelling and bruising?

Count on it. Almost everyone comes out of a face-lift with a swollen face. Some patients have very little, others more. In some cases, the facial features are distorted by the swelling. But it subsides quickly, especially if you keep your head elevated during the night and use a lot of cold compresses during the day.

Bruising usually doesn't appear until a day or two after surgery. Then it usually follows a progression over two to three weeks. The bruises start out a scary blue/purple color and fade to green, then yellow.

Here's a tip: Wait until day five after surgery, and then put warm compresses on the bruised areas. Use cold compresses for swelling on days one to five, and then warm compresses for bruising after day five.

What if I can't sleep?

Keeping your head elevated at night for the first few days to prevent excessive swelling doesn't go hand in hand with deep, restful sleep. Expect erratic sleep for a few days. But this too will pass. If it's really troubling, you may use a sleep aid (such as Ativan) for a few days.

Will there be scars?

Yes, but nobody will notice. You can't make an incision in the skin without leaving scars, but those scars are almost imperceptible. Incisions are usually made in areas that aren't readily noticeable. For face-lifts, they're mainly around the ears and into the hairline. Complete healing can take anywhere from a few months to a year.

How safe is it?

Statistically, it's safer than driving your car with respect to major complications.

What are the risks?

Complications can include excessive bleeding, infection, and poor healing. These are rare. Rarer complications include bad reactions to the anesthesia, leading to lung and heart trouble. There's a remote chance of blood clots that can travel to the heart or brain, causing heart attack or stroke. Neurological reactions to either the anesthesia or the surgery could lead to nerve damage. A thorough medical pre-screening will reduce the risk of such complications.

When is the best time for a face-lift?

The best time is when you've been concerned about your appearance for some time. If you're like most of my patients, you won't do it on the spur of the moment. You'll have thought long and hard about it.

How long will I be off work?

You can usually go back to work in two weeks. However, if you're worried about your "coming out," take three weeks to be sure. With "mini" lifts, the healing is about one week faster.

Will I be in the hospital?

Some plastic surgeries are performed in hospitals. You might stay overnight or be sent home the same day. Many surgeries are performed in private clinics. In accredited clinics, the operating rooms are equipped in the same way as found in hospitals.

What procedures must be done before surgery?

You'll need to go through the basic preparations you would go through for any surgery. These include a complete physical examination by your family doctor, including blood tests, an electrocardiogram, and X-rays, where indicated.

You'll be asked many questions about your health and lifestyle. It's important to be completely forthright. Your answers are important to your surgeon and anesthesiologist (who will put you to sleep and monitor your condition throughout the operation).

What kind of anesthetic will I have?

For most surgeries on the face, expect either a general anesthetic or a local, "twilight," or neuroleptic anesthesic. Much of this decision is based upon the surgeon's experience, the medical facilities, the length and type of your procedure, and your wishes. An anesthesiologist will administer a combination of drugs and constantly monitor your progress throughout the surgery. These drugs take time to wear off, so you may feel a little disoriented or nauseated afterward.

Will people know I've "had work"?

Not unless you tell them. Most patients report getting compliments on how young and fresh they look, followed by questions on what brought about this transformation. These include questions about weight loss, a new exercise regimen, or a change in wardrobe or hairstyle.

THE CONSULTATION

Consultations usually consist of two stages.

First Consultation
- The patient discusses his or her concerns.
- The doctor advises the patient of his or her options (both surgical and nonsurgical).
- The doctor determines if the patient is a good candidate for plastic surgery.
- Both the patient and doctor determine if they have a rapport.
- The doctor takes photographs for use in the next consultation and during surgery.

Second Consultation
- This is the planning session.
- It often involves the assistant surgeon, patient care coordinator, and clinic nurse.
- The photos taken during the initial consultation are used to show how the face-lift will proceed.
- The surgery date is set, and postoperative care is discussed.
- The patient signs a consent form stating that he or she understands what will happen and knows the risks (however small) of complications.

GIVING A MEDICAL HISTORY

When giving a medical history, you'll be asked for details by your family doctor, the clinic nurse, and the anesthesiologist. Some questions will be repeated at different stages. Here, you have to be patient and fully candid. Your answers are important. You'll be asked about the following:
- Medicines you're taking or have taken in the past, even over-the-counter pain relievers or cold remedies

– Allergies and family history of disease; if your mom had a stroke or your dad had a heart attack, we would like to know
– Whether you have a tendency to bleed excessively
– Drinking, smoking, and recreational drug use, now and in the past

Be honest. Nobody's judging you, and these questions have no wrong answers. You won't necessarily be ruled out because of your lifestyle, but advance knowledge on the part of the surgeon and anesthesiologist is key to avoiding surprises on the operating table.

PREPARING FOR THE FACE-LIFT

Marking the Skin

The plastic surgeon will mark the landmarks of your face with a surgical pen. These may include the following:

~ a dot for the midline point on the chin
~ another dot for the highest point on the cheekbone
~ a line along the jaw
~ another line down each side of the neck
~ lines on the folds that fall from each side of the nose and mouth
~ an arc across each side of the mid-face
~ V-shaped marks for each of the two flat muscles in the front of the neck
~ incision lines as reference points, which indicate the path around each ear, across the temple hair, and back into the hairline

Anesthesia

Prior to being given general anesthesia, the patient is given an intravenous drip (e.g., a potassium-sodium compound) to keep him or her hydrated during surgery. The operating room nurse attaches a number of monitors to the patient, including a blood pressure cuff, electrocardiogram, and pulse oxymeter (which measures the heartbeat and oxygen levels in the blood).

Finally, an oxygen mask is placed over the patient's mouth and nose. As the patient takes a couple of deep breaths, the anesthetic is administered. It usually consists of three drugs:
- one to put the patient to sleep
- one to ensure that the patient feels no pain
- one to keep the patient from moving during surgery

Anti-nausea medication is often added during the procedure. Once the patient is asleep, a tube is inserted into the throat, which will carry oxygen and anesthetic gases that keep him or her asleep. Vital signs—blood pressure, heart rate, oxygen level in the blood—are monitored to ensure that the patient is adequately asleep, has enough pain relief, and is getting enough oxygen. Local anesthetic combined with adrenaline is injected into the patient's face and neck to constrict the blood vessels, reducing bleeding during surgery. Local intravenous sedation anesthesia is much the same except no tube is placed in the throat and no drugs to decrease movement are given.

THE FACE-LIFT

Face-lifts have come a long way. Initially, there was a skin-only lift. The skin was freed from the underlying tissue and pulled taut, with the excess skin trimmed away. This left tension on the skin and often resulted in that tight look that announced itself as a face that had gone under the knife.

Now the "lift" in face-lift is done not on the skin but on the *fascia*, the underlying tissue of the face. There are many ways to do this. Different surgeons have also coined many different terms to describe the various types of lifts, but most are variations of the following procedures.

Short Flap Lift

In its simplest form, small J-shaped incisions are made around the ears, allowing the fascia of the mid-face to be pulled up and sewn in place. It's usually called the "short flap," "short scar," or "J-flap" lift because of the size and shape of the incisions. Some plastic surgeons have trendy names for the short flap procedure, such as the Weekend Lift or Manhattan Lift (because it's popular in New York City). This kind of lift may be fine for younger patients who need a small amount of lift along the jawline.

Note: The Weekend Lift is a complete misnomer. There's no such thing, even if it's a long holiday weekend and you've taken an extra day. You can't have a procedure done on Friday and expect to be back to normal on Monday or Tuesday.

Standard Face-lift

The standard face-lift is similar to the short flap lift. The area lifted extends farther down the face into the neck area and deeper into underlying tissue. This face-lift is often referred to as SMAS (a medical acronym for the superficial musculoaponeurotic system, the tissue beneath the facial skin).

Deep Plane Face-lift

The deep plane face-lift is the standard lift taken a step further. It goes deeper into the face, elevating not only the skin but also the SMAS. It's a more technical procedure because it means working right on top of the facial nerves. But it allows the surgeon to get about double the lift. There are several safe modifications of this very effective lift.

Endoscopic Lift

An endoscopic lift, especially of the cheek or mid-face region, is done through small incisions in the temple. It's faster and simpler, but it isn't for everyone. An endoscopic procedure, such as the J-flap lift, may work well for a younger patient, but probably not for someone older.

Threading

Threading is a recent technique in cosmetic facial surgery, and simpler than a deep plane face-lift. Nylon threads with little barbs are inserted into the face and pulled taut. There are usually four or five on each side. Sometimes they're even placed in the forehead. However, the results haven't been that good overall, and very few, if any, of these procedures are being performed now.

Many excellent types of face-lift procedures are available today. By sharing your specific concerns about your face and neck with us, we can recommend the various surgical options to achieve the best results. This may or may not include some removal of neck fat or tightening of neckbands. You and your surgeon will mutually determine what's best for you.

TIPS FROM FACE-LIFT PATIENTS

One of the keys to successful surgery is practical information, not just from the office but also from patients who've been there. Here are some tips from patients who have had face-lifts.

Milla

Here are a few things I believe were significant in my recovery process:

- Get down pillows (I got two) with jersey knit pillow cases. You spend a lot of time lying down.
- Stock up on bottled water (cases of twenty-four), and don't forget bendable drinking straws.
- Buy soft foods such as Jell-O and applesauce. Basically anything you can get through a quarter-inch opening between your lips is wonderful.
- The men's button-front cotton shirt is the choice dress code after surgery. I picked up a half dozen at Goodwill for $2 each, washed them, wore them, and, when finished, washed them again and gave them back to Goodwill. Now that's recycling.
- Baseball caps are a good thing for going outdoors during the first couple of weeks.

D.G.

For anyone considering this course of action, here are a few pointers from my adventure:

- I found February or March was a very good time to drop out of sight for a couple of weeks.
- Be prepared. Have a good friend on standby at home.

- Stock up on straws, fluids, and totally soft foods. I lived on baby foods, yogurt, cream puddings, and, later, baked potato, well-mashed, with tinned salmon.
- Get your hair color done before, but don't get an extreme haircut. For a while, you may want to hide in your hair.
- Don't be dismayed if you upchuck the day after the anesthetic. Think of it as slimming.
- Be ready with button-up-the-front tops for a while.
- Look forward to enjoying the results, but don't be impatient.

Sylvia
When I lost weight, I received a great suggestion to indulge myself with chocolate pudding. I did—usually at 10 o'clock in the morning. Decadent!

Marta
Five days before the surgery, I had my hair cut very short and lightened by a shade. After the surgery, when I met extended family, friends, or acquaintances, they all made similar comments: "You look so good! You've cut your hair."

Mary K.
Change your hair; comb it over your ears to cover the surgery scars. Wear glasses to cover the puffiness around your eyes.

Judith
I had the vacation of my life! Not something you'd expect to hear post-surgery, is it? As it happens, stress management plays an important role in my professional practice, and to this end, I

offer guided imagery, hypnotherapy, and various techniques to induce and facilitate deep states of relaxation.

Well, with post-surgery instructions to rest, keep ice water compresses on my eyes, and stay put for a few days, I decided to give myself a generous dose of my own medicine. For four days, I kept the phone ringer off; ate and drank my carefully planned, nutrition-dense cleansing and detoxifying concoctions; meditated; traveled through umpteen guided imageries; and went in and out of self-induced trance. In between "sessions," I day-dreamed to Beethoven and Kreisler while my eyes rested under those blessedly soothing ice water compresses.

What a marvelous few days; I just floated on a feeling of well-being, all the while following doctor's orders.

CHAPTER NINE

Wisdom doesn't necessarily come with age.
Sometimes age just shows up all by itself.

– *Tom Wilson*, actor, writer, and comedian

BONITA'S GRADUATION

GRADUATION DAY

The time: late June. The place: a school auditorium just outside of Toronto.

Onstage, eighth-grade graduates are dressed in their best outfits and bubbling with preadolescent energy, getting ready to move onto high school.

In the crowded hall, amid proud parents, doting relatives, and supportive friends, Bonita, age fifty-seven, is having her own ceremony. Her mood is decidedly different. "I was so self-conscious," she recalls.

Twenty-one days earlier, Bonita was on the operating table, unconscious for more than three hours. She was going through a long-postponed face- and neck-lift. Her granddaughter's graduation is her first time in public. This is Bonita's "coming out party," and she's nervous.

Her face is still slightly swollen with traces of yellowish bruising, more on the left side than on the right. But that's not unusual. There isn't always a neat symmetrical progression to how face-lift patients heal. But she's coming to the end of her post-face-lift "rainbow days." That's when your bruised face seems to go through most of the colors in the rainbow—from blue to purple to green to yellow.

Bonita's discomfort isn't from the surgery. In her mind's eye, she sees herself as far more bruised and battered than she actually looks. She glances around nervously, certain that all eyes are on her and that people will ask if she's been mugged. No one does. Her husband, Don, tells her to relax.

BEFORE THE FACE-LIFT

Bonita is a classic beauty. She's tall and fair-haired with large, widely spaced, blazing blue eyes and high cheekbones. But, in recent years, Bonita's age has begun to show on her face. She has developed *ptosis*, medical terminology for drooping. Over the years, gravity has been working against her.

The eyes are the first thing you notice when you look at someone. If your eyes look tired, so will you. In Bonita's case, she had bags under her eyes. The ptosis also went to work on her nose and mouth, turning once-delicate lines into deepening furrows. But it didn't stop there. Bonita's face was moving south and finding a new home in her neck. There's no delicate way to put this: Bonita has developed turkey wattles.

Bonita thought about cosmetic surgery on and off for a few years. "I had a lot of those moments where you look in the mirror, realize that things are definitely not okay, and tell yourself that you've got to do something," she says. "But I always stopped short of taking action."

Bonita finally launched Operation Face-lift at the urging of husband Don. "He was the key factor," Bonita says. "He didn't actually say that I needed it, but he knew I thought that I needed it, so he pushed me to make the appointment."

THE CONSULTATION

Bonita comes in for her initial consultation. We discuss her concerns. She strikes me as a good candidate for cosmetic surgery—well-motivated and likely to have an excellent outcome. Bonita, in turn, feels confident in me. We've developed a rapport.

Bonita decides to go ahead. We take some photographs—full-face, three-quarter profile, full profile, and low-angle. They would be used at the next consultation and during surgery.

Bonita then goes to her family doctor for a checkup to make sure she's in overall good health. This includes blood tests, an electrocardiogram, and many questions about her health and lifestyle.

Bonita returns for her second consultation. This is the planning session, which is conducted by the doctor who assists me during and after surgery. Also present is our patient care coordinator and clinic nurse. We use the photos to show Bonita how we would proceed. We set a date for surgery and talk about postoperative care. Bonita gives us the green light to go ahead and signs the consent form.

SURGERY DAY

The big day arrives. Bonita, with Don at her side, comes to the clinic. The nurse takes her into the change room and helps her

into a gown and slippers. Don is told he should return in about
three hours. Like many concerned spouses, he sets up camp in
the waiting room. He isn't going anywhere.

Now, just before the nurse takes her into the operating
room, Bonita and I have our final preoperative meeting. It provides me with the opportunity to offer reassurance—and a last
chance for Bonita to change her mind. She doesn't, even though
she's plainly nervous.

We begin by marking the landmarks of Bonita's face with a
surgical pen. After I make all of my reference points, her face
looks like a road map.

The nurse guides Bonita into the operating room. Dr. Litner
is already there, as are the operating room nurse and anesthesiologist, Dr. Pam Goldberg. Bonita hasn't had anything to eat or drink
since the previous evening because she's going under general anesthetic. Like most patients, Bonita is worried about this issue, even
though she's been briefed ahead of time. The "What if?" factor is
still present.

Dr. Goldberg asks more of the now-familiar questions.
She wants to know if Bonita has had any unpleasant reactions,
such as nausea, from previous anesthetics. She replied that she
hasn't.

Bonita is placed on the table and covered with a heated
blanket. Dr. Goldberg secures an intravenous drip in her fore-
arm while the operating room nurse sets up monitors—a blood
pressure cuff, electrocardiogram leads, and a pulse oxymeter.
The nurse places a "stress ball" in each of Bonita's hands;
they're something to squeeze and serve as stress relievers to
help Bonita take her mind off the intravenous needle. The nurse

also holds Bonita's hand, providing a powerful and calming focal point.

Dr. Goldberg starts an intravenous drip, a potassium-sodium compound to keep Bonita hydrated. She places an oxygen mask over Bonita's mouth and nose and asks her to take a couple of deep breaths, filling the lungs with oxygen. Once Bonita does this, Dr. Goldberg starts the anesthetic.

The sleep-inducing drug is added to the intravenous line, along with anti-nausea medication. Dr. Goldberg, standing at Bonita's head, tells her that she may feel a slight burning in her arm. The aim here is to have no surprises for Bonita. As the drug takes effect, Dr. Goldberg tells her that when she wakes up, the operation will be over.

Bonita drifts off within a minute. The last sense she loses is her hearing, so noise in the operating room is kept to a minimum. She's now unconscious and completely unaware of what's going on around her.

Once Bonita is asleep, Dr. Goldberg inserts a tube into the throat that would carry oxygen and anesthetic gases that keep her asleep. She then moves to her post at a bank of monitors near the foot of the operating table to monitor Bonita's vital signs.

We move on to "hairstyling." Bonita's blond locks are trimmed along a narrow path following the pre-marked incision lines. Then her head is draped. We then inject local anesthetic combined with adrenaline in Bonita's face and neck.

It's time to begin. We start with liposuction. I make tiny incisions under the chin and on each side of the face just below the ear and insert a canula (a slender tube) into each incision, moving it back and forth to free up the skin. Then the liposuction machine is connected, and a small amount of neck fat is vacuumed out. The aim isn't to take out every last bit of fat but to sculpt the neck.

We perform a modified deep plane face-lift on Bonita. I draw the scalpel along the incision lines, holding it like a fine paintbrush, applying just the right amount of pressure so that my incision goes just through the skin but not into the deeper structures. It has to be a smooth, elegant motion, like a painter's brushstroke. When the incision is carried into the hairline, I change the angle of the blade, keeping it parallel to the hair follicles to avoid damaging them.

Now it's time to gently raise the skin from the underlying tissue, revealing the area in which the "lift" part of the face-lift will occur. This is the critical part of the operation. The real lift isn't on the skin, though that's where you want to see the results, but on the deeper tissues. The fascia is pulled up. I draw it back up into the position it had been in ten or fifteen years before. Some is trimmed away. Then it's fixed in place with sutures. This is the most rewarding part of the face-lift. As I draw up that tissue, because the skin was attached, it all comes up too. We can now see the impact of the lift. We drape the elevated skin back in place. Dr. Litner takes measurements. We achieved 29 millimeters (about one and a quarter inches) of lift on the underside of Bonita's face.

We proceed with the delicate process of tailoring away the excess skin and sewing Bonita up with dozens of fine sutures. Some will be taken out four days after surgery. Many are dissolving sutures that remain in place and are eventually absorbed by the body. I return to the neck. Two neck muscles, which tend to drift with age, are drawn a little closer together and secured with several sutures. The incision beneath the chin is closed.

Dr. Goldberg begins dialing down the knockout drugs. It's time for Bonita to wake up. She does so within a few minutes and is immediately lucid. The whole procedure takes three hours and thirty-five minutes.

> As a beauty I'm not a great star.
> Others are handsomer far;
> But my face—I don't mind it
> Because I'm behind it;
> It's the folks out front that I jar.

— *Anthony Euwer*, artist

RECOVERY

Bonita spends an uncomfortable night in the clinic. Small drains behind each ear and pressure stockings on her legs prevent blot clots. She feels nauseated and a little disoriented from the anesthetic. There are no dressings on her face, allowing the night nurse to keep an eye on the incisions. It's hard to sleep.

Day 1

In the morning, the drains and stockings are removed, and Bonita's head is swathed in bandages. Don takes her home.

Day 4

Don brings Bonita back for a scheduled visit. She's moving slowly and feeling fragile. The head dressing comes off. Bonita looks like she's had about ten pro fights—puffy around the eyes and bruised around the ears. "I go up and down," she says, her words barely audible. "Right now, I feel lousy." She's mildly nauseated and thinks it's from the codeine-laced Tylenol 3s she's been taking. Her face feels tight.

Bonita says her son won't visit because "he doesn't want to see me like this." Right now, the question of whether it was worth it is up for serious debate. Bonita is given some reassurance and is told that she's through the worst of it, her incisions are healing well, and she'll start to look fairly presentable in a week.

Bonita lies on the examining table, and the stitches under her chin and in front of her ears are removed. With each, there's a little pinch and much anxiety. She allows the tension to drain down her arms and into soft beanbag balls she holds in each hand.

Her head dressing is replaced with an inelegant but practical Lycra head and neck bandage. She can take it off to bathe; otherwise, it will stay on, day and night, for two weeks. Bonita is given a list of postoperative instructions and sent home.

Postoperative Tips

Do . . .	Do not . . .
– Drink a lot of fluids (not alcohol) and avoid hard-to-chew foods.	– Smoke for at least two weeks.
Do . . .	Do not . . .
– Keep your head elevated, as lying flat may increase swelling. Try sleeping on your back with two pillows under your head. – Keep cold compresses over ears, jaws, and neck (for at least twenty minutes every two hours) to help prevent excessive swelling. – Clean incisions two or three times a day. Apply Polysporin ointment to keep them moist. – Be gentle with the toothbrush (or use your finger). – Be careful around rambunctious children and restless bedmates. They could accidently bump your face.	– Bend over or lift anything heavier than five pounds. – Go outside in the sun without using a 30+ sunblock. – Get into a hot tub for a few weeks. – Take anything with aspirin in it, as it may cause bleeding.

Day 8

Bonita is back for another scheduled visit. She looks and feels much better. "I've had a couple of rough days, but overall it's been a good week," she reports. All remaining stitches are removed. Bonita asks about a tiny fold of skin behind one ear and is told that it will subside with time. Husband Don is at her side. He's been her home nurse, cleaning her stitches and applying Polysporin. "I don't know what I'd do without him," Bonita says.

Day 14

Bonita takes off the Lycra head dressing. She doesn't have to wear it any longer. Most, but not all, of the swelling and bruising have disappeared. She returns to work, still a little puffy. People tell her she looks great. She's grateful but takes it with a grain of salt. Bonita is their boss. The real test, she believes, will come when she ventures out in public among strangers.

Day 21

Bonita attends her granddaughter's graduation.

Day 56

It's been eight weeks since her surgery. Bonita feels back to normal and looks like a younger version of her old self. She and Don celebrate with a trip to Hawaii. The swelling has subsided, and the rainbow of bruises has vanished.

Day 90

Bonita's face still feels a little numb in places. That, too, isn't unusual. Some numbness can persist for up to a year. She's "still not 100 percent" but feels good about herself. "I look ten years younger," she says.

Day 113

It has now been four-and-a-half months since the surgery. Bonita returns for her second-to-last checkup. She's healed well. The fold of skin behind her ear has disappeared. Bonita is brimming with health and energy. She says, "I used to look in the mirror a lot and say to myself, 'That's not good.' Now I still look in the mirror a lot and say, 'That's great.'"

The difficult day or so immediately after surgery is now just a blur. "Looking back on it, I remember feeling tired, but I don't remember any pain," she reports. She also says people are complimenting her on her fresh, youthful appearance.

CHAPTER TEN

Time is a great healer, but a poor beautician.

— *Lucille S. Harper,* columnist

MARGUERITE'S UPLIFTING EXPERIENCE

Nobody should rush into plastic surgery. Marguerite thought long and hard about it before deciding to go ahead with her face-lift. She came in for an initial consultation, went home to give it some more thought, and didn't return for a year. She kept this diary of her experience.

-1-

Change Sets In

A couple of years ago, I somehow lost five kilograms (about twelve pounds) while trekking in the Andes. It improved my figure but had a reverse impact on my face, which looked more drawn. I'd gracefully accepted the squaring of my lower jaw over the years. But now new heavy parentheses framed my mouth. Fine vertical lines ran from my lips, draining out whatever lipstick I put on. It gave my mouth an aging look. I never had many wrinkles. My problem was the change in my face from the nice oval of the young face to a more square shape—and the sagging. My problem was due to time and the pull of gravity.

At the very time when I was trying to cope with my "new old look," the media obsessed about "cosmetic rejuvenation" for baby boomers. Many relatively new nonsurgical procedures were available for a promising "lunchtime face-lift." I had heard about surgical procedures that promised quick recovery. It was all very tempting.

The quickie doesn't exist. You won't be returning to your normal life after just a few days. Everybody wants a rapid recovery, but even with the most minimal face-lift, it's hard to imagine that anyone can look good after just a few days. For one thing, wait at least four days before having the stitches taken out. If you take them out any sooner, the wounds can open up. After three or four days, you could put a kerchief on and go out to the store for some milk and bread—but that's about it.

Almost all surgical procedures in the face will take at least a week to ten days—at the short end—before you'll feel sociable. Usually, it's two to three weeks.

-2-

A Consultation

It does get me to thinking about doing something with my "beauty marks," especially the lower one, which didn't appear until my twenties. I'm so used to them that I tend to forget they're there.

*From time to time, toddlers, with their brutal frank-
ness, poke at them, asking, "What's this?" I then have to
explain to them that they're my beauty marks. That's why I
am beautiful. They remain puzzled and unconvinced. However, I had recently met someone who did get turned on by
my moles—at first. For his sake, I have to put any idea of
removing them on the back burner for the time being.*

*I'm lucky. Dr. Adamson has a cancellation. Instead of
waiting three months, I have my consultation with him in
just a few days.*

*He carefully explains that there are three levels to con-
sider in the face: the underlying bone structure (nothing
wrong with mine), the layer of muscles and tissues, and,
lastly, the skin.*

*Dr. Adamson outlines the benefits of a rhytidectomy, a
face- and neck lift, which will give me "a more refined jaw,
smoother neck, and contoured cheeks." Gently pulling my
cheeks out and upward, he shows me the expected results in
the mirror.*

*He goes through a long list of dreadful possible effects
of the rhytidectomy, most with a fairly low possibility of
one in 10,000. (But what if you're the one?) The literature
from his office also refers to "some discomfort."*

*For the mouth area, he recommends a non-permanent
injection of the filler Restylane. My upper mole has a round
and fairly large base. Its excision would leave a visible scar.
Dr. Adamson would prefer simply shaving off both moles,
which are dark brown and protruding, leaving a flat base in
a lighter skin color. I like the idea.*

I always ask patients when they come in exactly what it is that bothers them. Marguerite said that gravity was increasing the folds that come down from the corner of the nose and giving her jowls and lines that we (not very delicately, I guess) call "drool lines." Those are the furrows at the corner of the mouth. She told me she was ambivalent about her birthmarks.

I thought she was pretty committed to going ahead. I make notes about how committed I feel people are, and I put her down at 70 percent, which means that I thought there was a 70 percent probability that, after seeing me that first day, she would indeed go ahead with surgery. I felt she had reasonable goals and expectations, had thought about it, and had the personality and character to go through with it satisfactorily.

-3-

Mixed Feelings

I'm left pondering whether I'd have the courage to endure the pain and take the risk of complications. Can I be sufficiently self-centered to squander on cosmetics funds that could feed a good number of Bolivian children for a whole year? In the meantime, the world has turned more chaotic than ever with 9/11. I feel some guilt getting involved in such mundane concerns.

The new man in my life professes to like women who are "a little vain." It soon becomes clear that the emphasis is on "little." He would be totally aghast if I mentioned my plans.

My daughter is vehemently against it. She's the type of person who likes everything to be natural, so something like this is very, very bad from her point of view. I guess at her age, twenty-nine, she doesn't understand.

The few friends with whom I bring up the subject are quite supportive. They show much interest in witnessing my example to see if they would like to follow suit. Once, when I was visiting my sister, a friend of hers remarked that I looked young for my age and wondered if it was thanks to a face-lift. My sister exclaimed that I'd never do such a thing. I was too au naturel for that. Well, that was five years ago. With my impending sixtieth birthday, perhaps I've changed.

Months go by until I feel ready to seriously consider the matter. There is no longer a man in my life—one fewer considerations to deal with. I go back to Dr. Adamson a year to the day after my first visit.

Marguerite had many written questions on her second visit. She wrote down all my responses. She's an engineer, so it fits her character to be a fact finder, think about it for a good long time, and then make a decision.

-4-
Setting It Up

Dr. Adamson goes over my file and tells me that my propensity to bruising may delay recovery by a couple of days but doesn't present a problem. The hairs growing from the moles may disappear when the moles are shaved off, depending on how deep the follicles are. The advantage of a temporary filler such as Restylane around the mouth is that it would give me a chance to see if I like the look. We discuss laser treatments to reduce lines around the mouth.

I then go over administrative details with Deborah, who offers me a surgery date a month hence. It sounds good; enough time to prepare myself but not so much that I'd start losing my momentum. It also fits my schedule perfectly. I know if I don't grab it, I'll have to wait at least another three months and work myself up to it once more. I ask Deborah to have a couple of former patients with profiles similar to mine call me.

Dr. Adamson's associate, Dr. Bagal, goes over the details of the surgery process, a fairly long list of possible complications (the ultimate being death). She gives me a number of prescriptions for antibacterials and antivirals as well as Tylenol 3 to ease post-surgery "discomfort."

I'm asked simply to sign an acknowledgment that I've been apprised of the horrendous complications that may arise (albeit with a relatively low possibility) rather than a waiver, as I had expected.

During my next visit the following week, he tells me more about laser treatment versus fillers. The laser will clear up fine vertical lines, what I aim for, while fillers are aimed more at changing the mouth shape, giving it a fuller, sexier look. I guess it's something like sandblasting versus tuckpointing.

I finally decide to have the laser treatment at the same time as the face-lift. Financially and psychologically, it's more efficient. I have to take exfoliants and demelanizing agents for a couple of weeks prior to treatment.

Dr. Adamson takes mug shots: full face, left and right semi-profiles, and profiles.

One of the most important things anyone considering plastic surgery can do is to talk to people who've had it done. Some will be eager to discuss every detail; others won't. But a conversation with someone who's been there will always help.

Marguerite will have a face-lift. Two facial moles will be shaved off, and she'll have some laser resurfacing to reduce deep vertical lines around her mouth. For this, she must prepare her skin with exfoliants and demelanizing agents. This involves applying cream that produces a mild facial peel, along with mild skin bleach, and a steroid cream. There can be side effects, as Marguerite discovers.

-5-

Preparations and Complications

The month up to surgery day goes quickly. I meet with two former patients, one for lunch, the other for coffee. A year after their surgeries, they don't recall clearly the details of what they went through, something akin to labor pains and having a baby. Memory can be selective. One mentions that she still has at times a feeling of tightness around the jaw. They're both very positive about the whole experience and satisfied with their results. They do much to allay my fears.

On the basis of their experience and after consulting with Dr. Adamson's office, I arrange a private nurse who'll come home with me the morning after the operation and spend a few hours making sure I'm all right on my own.

My family doctor gives me a complete physical. I also get blood work, an electrocardiogram, and a chest X-ray.

A professional photographer takes portraits from all angles, to be used as a guideline during surgery.

Two weeks before surgery I dutifully stop taking any vitamin that may be a blood thinner. At bed-time, I start applying the exfoliating and demelanizing agents around the mouth. Within a couple of days, the whole area has turned red. Another couple of days, and I have to take Tylenol to dull the pain so I can sleep at night. By the end of the week, I can't bear it anymore and call the office.

Dr. Bagal promptly returns my call. I'm told to stop the exfoliant for a couple of days to give the skin a rest and return to it in the days just preceding the operation. It seems to work, with the help of yet more Tylenol.

I haven't told any of the friends with whom I discussed it a year earlier of my decision—nor anyone else, for that matter. My daughter was overseas. I wasn't even going to tell her, but because she had a major earthquake in her life at that time, she unexpectedly came back. It was three weeks before the operation. I tell her about it, and she agrees to spend the weekend with me after the operation, which is scheduled for a Thursday. Since I had made up my mind, she was supportive.

The most common error made in matters of appearance is the belief that one should disdain the superficial and let the true beauty of one's soul shine through. If there are places on your body where this is a possibility, you are not attractive — you are leaking.

— Fran Lebowitz, **author**

-6-

The Day Before

Getting ready takes me the whole day before the operation. I set up camp downstairs, making my bed on the living room sofa to avoid going up and down stairs to feed myself. I gather firm and oversized cushions to keep me propped up while resting and sleeping to avoid swelling.

I tape Dr. Adamson's telephone number to all the phones in the house so that if I needed to call (and, as it turned out, I did), I wouldn't have to look for it.

I cook up a storm: gallons of chicken stock, beef stew, muffins, strawberries poached in syrup, apple compote, and stewed prunes. I stock up on yogurt, juice, and tea. There's enough nice mushy food in the fridge and freezer to hold for a week without having to go out.

-7-

Surgery Day

When morning arrives, I put on a dress that buttons all the way down, take nothing but my house keys, and

*simply go by subway to Dr. Adamson's clinic, across the
street from his office.*

*The elevator brings me to the second floor, where I
enter a reception room, which could be that of any fancy
downtown corporation. It's elegantly furnished. The walls
are decorated with prints by Matisse, and soothing background music filters through a sound system.*

*The operating room nurse, a big smile on her face, wel-
comes me, and takes me first to the (un)dressing room. I feel
that, no matter what happens from here on, she could carry
me off to safety. With the gown I get slippers to keep my feet
warm. This is a far cry from the atmosphere of the public
health system. Even the OR feels as relaxing as a lounging
area as I lie on the operating table under a nice heated blanket.*

*Dr. Un, the anesthesiologist, comes in, cracking a joke.
The only time I'd had general anesthesia was half a century
ago for an appendectomy. A chloroform mask was put on my
face and sent me under before I could count to ten, as
requested. He tells me that things indeed have changed. I'm
going to get an intravenous "champagne cocktail." The intravenous is plugged in. Unfortunately, I won't even get high.*

*Dr. Adamson joins us. It's only 9:30, but he's already
done a blepharoplasty (eyelid surgery). Dr. Bagal is here as
well—and who else? I can't remember. . . .*

*4:00 p.m.: I wake up in the recovery room. I must
have been here for a couple of hours. I'm somehow propped
up in a reclining chair. Blankets are folded from both sides
of the chair toward me. There's no footrest, and I keep slid-
ing down. Every time I prop myself back up a sharp pain*

shoots through my head. I'm too hot, then too cold; I spread out the covers, then bring them back together, not knowing how to tuck myself in this unfamiliar bedding arrangement. I have no recollection of the afternoon recovery room nurse.

The night nurse, Nurse Angel, commiserates at every groan I utter, telling me how difficult the first night is but that everything will be all right later on. She patiently helps me to slide back up on the chair. She wipes my forehead with a damp cloth. I could adopt her as my mother. In the early morning, she walks me to the bathroom, where she gives me a shower and washes my hair.

-8-
Day 1: The Zombie Look

Shortly before the 7 a.m. discharge time, Dr. Bagal comes in to examine me. The operation went well. My head is gener- ously wrapped all around in white gauze. It's the zombie look. The swelling, combined with the dressing, seem to double my head's volume. Nurse Angel urges me not to look in mirrors for a while. Together with my private nurse, who arrived a while ago, they wheel me through to the ele- vator and down to the indoor garage where a town car is waiting to whisk me home.

My private nurse is prim, proper, and pretty. She expertly organizes my medication, bandages, and toiletry and gets me to slurp some food through my tight lips. Com- fortably propped up in the sofa bed of the living room, and with something finally in my stomach after a day-and-a- half-long fast, I start to feel much better. My private nurse sits by my side the whole morning, pampering me while I drift in and out and shake off the anesthetic and the shock from surgery.

By the end of her four-hour shift, we agree that I have all I need handy and will be just fine on my own. It takes me the whole afternoon to read the paper, in between naps, soft snacks, drinks, and swallowing Tylenol.

By evening, my daughter arrives to spend the long weekend with me. I've warned her not to gasp at the sight of me. Faced with a fait accompli, she turns out to be very supportive, just teasing me a bit about her "mummy mommy." She has some difficulty understanding how one could submit to such self-injury.

The weekend turns into a pyjama party. We watch videos. On Saturday, I manage to open my mouth suffi-ciently to brush my teeth. It does feel good. Showering isn't a problem as long as I'm careful to keep my head dry.

-9-

Day 4: Bandages Off

On the morning of day four, a town car comes to collect me for my second checkup. After some misleading hand ges-tures, the chauffeur parades my enormous bandaged head around his car for all the neighbors to see before finally tak-ing me downtown.

Nurse Maureen expertly removes the white bulky dressing to replace it with an elastic flesh-colored bandage, which wraps with Velcro on top of the head and at the back of the neck. I can now cover my head and go about without

*looking like a zombie. I drive my daughter to the bus sta-
tion and drop her off.*

*Later that afternoon, as I remove the bandage to mas-
sage my chin and ears with Polysporin, the chin starts to
bleed. I feel faint and lie down for two hours before feeling
able to call the office. Nurse Maureen calls back promptly
and reassures me. She'll call again in the evening to make
sure I'm all right.*

*A couple of days later, I muster the courage to go out,
hidden behind sunglasses and under a scarf, and run some
errands. No one stares at me.*

-10-

Day 8: The Swelling Goes Down

*Eight days after surgery, at my next checkup, Nurse Mau-
reen adroitly and painlessly removes my sutures. I'm finally
allowed to gently wash my hair without scratching the
scalp. It's a great relief. The Polysporin, together with resi-
due from the surgery and the natural accumulation of oil,
has made it disgustingly slimy.*

*Swelling on the left side of the face has now gone
down (my moon face of the past week had a lopsided shape).*

*Both ears are sticking out, with my shoulder-length
hair stubbornly splitting on either side. The laser treatment
has left a pinkish mask around the mouth area.*

*The lips are swollen. The cheeks feel like an endless
expanse of wood and plaster, numb except for some tingling
and a sensation of heat as blood flow and nerve connections
resume.*

A seesaw sensation runs up and down behind the ears, with a shooting sharp pain from time to time.

My allotted supply of Tylenol 3 runs out, but I can now manage with over-the-counter Tylenol. Tired of being cooped up at home, I venture to a movie theater, checking to make sure nobody I know is around.

-11-

Day 12: Camouflage Makeup

On the twelfth day after surgery, the makeup artist comes to my place to demonstrate camouflage makeup. She carefully selects and tests a tone of "Professional Secrets" foundation, one shade darker than my natural skin tone. She demonstrates how to apply a good layer on the area to be concealed by gentle patting and how to just spread for a lighter coat on the rest of the face. A light face powder will then ensure that the foundation stays on for the whole day. She also gets me to put on some blushing powder and lipstick to distract attention from critical areas of the face. With my endless wooden cheeks, white face, and blobs of rouge, I look like a cross between a china doll and some strange Western geisha.

I'm now ready for my first business meeting the following day. The person I'm dealing with doesn't recognize me at first. It must be the hat, scarf, and sunglasses.

The bruising, which had spread from the neck to just above the breast, is now practically gone, after going through various colors of the rainbow. I no longer have to sleep with my head elevated. I can even sleep on my side.

The invisible strangler who got hold of my neck two weeks ago has now released his grip. I can even chew and eat regular food.

-12-
Day 18: A Makeup Crisis

The time to return to a regular schedule has come. I'm scheduled to participate in an intensive, one-week study program. The damp heat that continues to prevail all week turns out to be truly oppressive in the rooms where the program is being held. There's no air conditioning. It leaves me exhausted.

"Professional Secrets" foundation and powder can't hold under the heat and humidity and turn into a plaster cake. More makeup comes off when I wipe my mouth after meals. I look like a mess by the end of each day. My study companions, all strangers at the beginning of the week, are sufficiently polite not to pay attention.

-13-
Day 21: No One Can Tell

At my three-week checkup, Nurse Maureen tells me the bandage must be worn one more week at night. She advises me to massage my cheeks and exercise the neck, which remains too stiff.

An overseas friend comes to visit for a couple of weeks. She's an early riser. I find it practically impossible to apply my "Professional Secrets" before sitting together for breakfast. She's shortsighted and doesn't notice the pink mask around the mouth or the missing moles, much less the face-lift.

Over the next two months, a number of people will comment on my long hair or tell me that I look well, but no one, not even the friend who heartily recommended I have them excised, will remark on my missing moles or other changes.

Eight weeks after surgery, my nephew comes to visit. On his second day here, he looks at me and asks me if I've lost weight. He obviously has noticed a change for the better but can't interpret it correctly.

-14-

Day 70: My Face Is My Own Again

My next checkup comes after two-and-a-half months. By that time, all the disjointed pieces of my face puzzle have fallen back into place. My face does belong to me again, the look not exactly younger, but rather, refreshed and relaxed. Staring at the mirror in the morning is no longer an ordeal.

The chin line is now well-defined. Crevasses on either side of the mouth have smoothed out. The fine lines running up and down from the lips have disappeared; I can apply lipstick without it being smudged into them. The cheek contour is much neater. My face looks lighter without the dark, protruding moles.

My only problems remain numbness on the sides just ahead of the ears and a recurring dampness in the ear canal, which I clean with Q-tips. Both Nurse Maureen and Dr. Adamson tell me that one should never put anything smaller than the elbow into the ear. Forget Q-Tips, and let nature take its self-cleaning course.

On an out-of-town trip, I go to visit a friend who had stayed at my place in the days just before the operation. Suddenly, she interrupts our animated conversation to ask me if I've had cosmetic surgery. Finally, someone with a keen sense of observation! I hug her.

A month later, I resume my facials. My aesthetician, who's regularly stood over every pore of my face for twenty years (and with whom I discussed cosmetic surgery at length eighteen months ago), doesn't bat an eyelash. They used to say "only her hairdresser knows for sure." Now, one could add "even her aesthetician doesn't know" (or rather won't tell as, in her experience, some of her clients don't wish to share such things afterward).

-15-
One Year Later: The New Real Me

A year later, I've now gone through my last checkup with Dr. Adamson. All aftereffects of the operation are totally gone. The new face is totally mine. I tend to forget I ever had the operation. I just enjoy this "new real me," the face in which I feel 100 percent comfortable and confident, the face I like to see reflected in the mirror every morning.

I enjoy being told that I look very well, much younger than my age and that I haven't changed in years. There's just one problem. I tend to be more observant of my friends' sagging chins and jowls. Why don't they . . . ?

CHAPTER ELEVEN

It has been almost a year since
I had cosmetic surgery.
Has my life changed? No,
but I sure feel wonderful.

— **Shirley**, patient

FABULOUS FACES

The emotional road map through cosmetic surgery usually begins somewhere around dissatisfaction and follows a route through uncertainty, fear, courage, and hope, eventually winding up at happiness. Tanya described her experience in six words: dreadful, hopeful, painful, cheerful, peaceful, and thankful.

The following patients describe their personal journeys and experiences with face-lifts.

NATASHA

I grew up realizing I am not conventionally beautiful or even particularly pretty, but I'd be cheered by friends and family saying I had a mobile, sympathetic face that did me well enough. But when I turned fifty, I spent time in front of the mirror with my fingertips, lifting my face back into a younger, less saggy position, wistfully wishing I looked better than I did.

I talked a lot with Suzanne, a trusted friend, and, reassured, I decided on a face-lift. She encouraged me to allow myself one cosmetic procedure and one alone, so I wouldn't become addicted to wanting more and more. It was very wise advice. My biggest fear was suffering nerve damage from the operation. I even feared it might happen as a kind of Godly judgment on my vanity.

I was glad to have avoided television programs on the procedure, which I have subsequently watched and know would certainly have put me off.

The ideas that helped me were that it isn't so different from having crowns on my teeth or dying the grey from my hair, and that I wouldn't look different—just "refreshed." This helped me feel I wasn't going to abnormal lengths to preserve my youth or avoid the inevitability of old age. I just wanted to go on looking like I was enjoying life.

After more reassurance, I got the operation.

The staff was endlessly cheerful and kind, and made the whole project feel normal. They respected my need for staying in the closet about the face-lift, except for a very few close friends. The nurse who was with me the first night was a saint. I can't imagine anyone more sympathetic or helpful.

The first postoperative night was tough, but every day from then on was better. I sat up in bed for the first days and nights at home with a bed rest contraption to keep my head elevated and the swelling down. The stitches all round my head made lying on my side too sore. My best friend brought me goodies as I listened to taped books and music— not a bad way to spend four or five days.

Three weeks after the operation, I was back at work with a spectacular new hairstyle to draw people's attention away from my new face. Amazingly, few people noticed anything, though I had a lot of comments about looking less tired.

So I look the same as I did before the operation, to myself and to others, except people now think I'm in my early forties. Strangely, I find I have more energy. What a bonus! I see myself a decade younger and behave as though I am.

I have no regrets at all—and, as yet, there has been no heavenly punishment.

Like it or not, society puts a premium on youth. Maintaining a youthful appearance has become especially important in the business world.

LIZ

How do I feel about my cosmetic surgery? I love it!

It's given me new vitality. Like it or not, when we look good, we feel good—at least, that's certainly the case for me. I've been motivated to lose thirty pounds since the surgery, and the compliments keep coming.

While I won't deny that my primary motivation was vanity, it was also driven by a need to stay competitive in my business. I work in a very young industry. My success almost totally depends on my ability to communicate with my customers. It's a lot easier when they relate to me more as an older colleague than as a friend of their mothers—and, for the record, my business is doing very well right now.

I'm simply a happier, rested, more relaxed-looking version of my former self—and every morning when I look in the mirror, it makes me smile.

The next two accounts come from two very different women, Sylvia and Valerie, both with "aging face" problems. Sylvia represents a departure from the usual way that people reach a decision to have cosmetic surgery. When she was fifty-one, her friends, family and family doctor nudged her towards getting a face-lift. Valerie made the decision herself at the tender age of seventy.

SYLVIA

When it was brought to my attention by my doctor that cosmetic facial surgery would work wonders, I laughed and went on with my life.

Several months later, I was told that I continuously look tired because of sagging eyelids. Other disturbing comments followed about my sagging chin and neck. People asked if I'd lost a lot of weight. I hadn't. I reported this to my husband, and he said that I was starting to show my age—fifty-one. Well, that was it! I was confused, frustrated, and frightened.

It's been one year now since my surgery. I look ten years younger, and I feel great about myself. It was a great self-esteem builder.

VALERIE

I can't tell you how good I've felt about myself this past year. When I look in the mirror, I see an attractive middle-aged woman instead of an older lady showing her age. My inner self and my outer self are now balanced and in harmony.

I'm thrilled each time I'm challenged on my senior citizen status and when friends remark, "Sylvia, how do you stay so young?" Recently, I attended a luncheon of my high-school girlfriends, and I know that I looked my best. That gave me a warm, fuzzy feeling.

For the two-week period of discomfort after the surgery, I knew that any information I needed was just a phone call away. If I had to make the decision again—face-lift, yes or no—you can bet the answer would be a resounding "yes."

After seventy years, I finally got up the nerve to do something just for me, and I have no regrets.

KATHERINE

Sometimes, the expression "Timing is everything" holds quite true. A chance photo in the middle of home renovations sent Katherine on her path toward cosmetic surgery.

As I approached my sixtieth year, life was good. Cosmetic surgery had crossed my mind several times in the past few years, but then I'd dismiss it. That was for later—sometime in the future. I felt young and energetic. We had a full schedule with travel, family, work, friends, art school, and home renovations.

A chance photo taken on a June holiday changed my mind. What a shock! Stop with the house! I need renovations! When I arrived home in July, I began to research the subject in earnest.

A website offered photos and explanations of various procedures, plus a list of plastic surgeons in Canada. I spoke to friends who had gone through the surgery and got the names of their doctors. Price, though important, wasn't the deciding factor. Qualifications, professionalism, and personality were. After all, this was my face, not some hidden body part. Dr. Adamson's qualifications and reputation in the community are very high. His involvement in humanitarian work in Russia was impressive, as was his list of accomplishments.

We met for an interview. I liked it—simple.

At a second interview several weeks later, the procedures were decided upon: face-, neck- and brow–lift, along with laser treatment.

The day finally arrived. My husband, Peter, drove me to the clinic, where we were greeted by two nurses and the anesthesiologist, all friendly, relaxed people. Imagine, if you can, after changing into a gown, walking on your own two legs into an operating room decorated with lively, colorful artwork, then hoisting yourself onto the table while chatting amiably.

In the two weeks of recovery, I had never spent so much time pampering myself. It was a novel experience to wake up in the morning and see what color was splashed across my face and watch the swelling subside. There was a kaleidoscope of color: a plum purple mouth that wandered on its own, a chartreuse neck, and, best of all, green eyes glittering in a sea of red. The shape of the mouth was interesting. Think fish lips.

I couldn't get my teeth to fit together. Soft foods were advised, so I lived on scrambled eggs and soup à la Peter and ice cream for the sore throat. I lost weight. Poor me. Ha!

I was unable to wear my hearing aids for two weeks because of the swelling around my ears. I was unable to talk on the phone, as my mouth refused to form words without lisping. I read, walked the dog when no one was about, watched TV, and listened to CDs and the stereo. The TV was so loud because of my lack of hearing that the poor dog left the room whining and wouldn't return until all was quiet once more.

One of the most delightful results of the surgery was Peter watching me closely every morning as the changes took place. Every day presented a new and different face. He was amazed.

At the end of the second week, most of the bruising had faded. Cheekbones appeared. My chin took shape. Some of the swelling was down. Best of all, the mouth I had known in younger days had returned.

Peter can't stop looking at me. After forty years of marriage, it's a pleasure to once more be the center of his attention and wonder. He can't stop grinning. I'm ecstatic!

Nanci and Daniel both had issues with inheritances that they wanted to give back to their parents.

NANCI

I've always felt uncomfortable with my double chin (okay, let's be honest: It was a triple). I came by it honestly; both my parents had multiple chins as well.

I hated photos of myself. I tried to position myself in business meetings so that others weren't looking at my profile. Weight loss and exercise didn't help enough, and aging was just making matters worse.

I made the decision to undergo a lower face- and neck lift with liposuction. It has now been more than six months since I had this done.

The change in my appearance was so subtle that no one who wasn't in the know had any idea that I'd undergone surgery. The only difference in my life is that I now receive a lot of compliments on my appearance. People ask me if I've lost weight or changed my hairstyle. Many remark on how great I look. I'm now delighted to have my picture taken.

DANIELLE

Dr. Adamson has robbed me of my heritage. My family has a strong tendency to develop jowls. At sixty-plus, after a long and happy association with my face, I realized my inheritance was starting to show up. I was developing those beside-the-mouth furrows, ending in a below-the-chin line droop. The rest of me was still quite presentable.

I asked my hairdresser if he'd noticed any good cosmetic work from his point of view (hairdressers are generally good scouts in this area). He reported that a couple of his clients had remarkable results from "some guy called Adamson."

I booked an initial consultation with Dr. Adamson and eventually had a lower face treatment that sent me home looking like the Woman in the Iron Chinstrap . . . and eventually looking fine—not younger, not sexier, just looking and feeling very nice.

Goodbye jowls!

MARY-ANNE

Mary-Anne was becoming one of the invisible people and wasn't happy about it. She decided to do something about it and is quite happy with the results.

I'm going to be fifty-one this year, and I look absolutely gorgeous.

Nine months ago, I had the works—my eyes, face, and neck. I did it for two reasons. The first was vanity, absolutely. The second was anger. I was getting very angry with society. Middle-aged ladies become invisible. You see it in how they treat you in restaurants. I hate it when they say "ma'am." It's not that I want preferential treatment; it's just that I want to stay in the game with the thirty-five-year-olds. Women in their mid-thirties have their pick of the

tables, and you're just told, "Okay, well, sit over there."
You notice it in how people bump into you in the street and
never say, "Sorry." It's as if you're not there. You see it in
business, and it's everywhere else. It's a youth-oriented soci-
ety. Middle-aged women have a tough time. I don't condone
it, but that's the way it is.

I was becoming one of those invisible people. My face
was starting to look old. My neck was really horrible, and
my upper eyelids seemed to be literally covering my eyes.
I'd put makeup on, and it would disappear. Sometimes you
have a better day and then you pay less attention to it, but
sometimes you say, "Okay, this is it. I have to do something
about it because society won't change."

Our iconic figures are from the world of entertain-
ment. It's a very shallow image to project. It's like cloning.
Everybody has to look the same. In Europe, there are all
kinds of shapes and sizes and forms and colors and every-
thing else, and they're still beautiful in their own way. But if
you live here, you do something to update your position.
That's the way I look at it.

I went to a doctor to see about getting something
done about the lines around my mouth. He used Botox
near my lip, and I looked like a stroke victim for about
a week and a half. I went back, and he said, "Oh well,
we'll use less the next time." So it wasn't a very pleasant
experience.

Then I saw my friend Philippa, who had just had her
eyes done, and she looked absolutely fantastic. So, one day
I woke up and said, "Okay, I'll make an appointment."

The doctor told me he would probably not be able to do a 100 percent improvement with my eyes, just maybe 80 percent. But 80 percent would be a fantastic result compared to what I had. So I definitely wanted my eyes done, and I felt I needed my neck done. He pointed out that the results would be different if I had a face-lift. It wasn't a sales job; he just matter-of-factly said it. If a professional points it out to you, you see it. And because the recovery time would be virtually the same, I said, "You know what? I'll probably never go under the knife again, so I might as well do it all at once."

Philippa came to pick me up the morning after the surgery, and I saw a shocked look on her face. It wasn't because I looked bad, but because she didn't see any change. Of course, I hadn't swollen up yet, but I had no bruising. For the first three days there was discomfort. You feel out of commission, and you're swollen. You feel like you're going to burst.

After five days, I was downtown doing my banking, wearing a head bandage and a hood. After eight days, I got a call from Deborah in the doctor's office to arrange for me to see the camouflage makeup artist. She asked, "Are they purple, or are they yellow?" (meaning my bruises). I said, "Well, gee, I have none." So I didn't get the camouflage makeup treatment.

I can tell exactly how many years this has taken off my face: eleven. I belong to a tennis club, and the girls at the reception desk are all young enough to be my granddaughters. I went in there and said, "If you can guess my age, I'll

*buy you dinner." And they said thirty-nine. This has been
fantastic. No one has put me over forty.*

*After seven weeks, I went on a blind date with a surgeon, and he couldn't tell a damn thing. He's not a cosmetic
surgeon, but he's still a surgeon who can tell stitches, and
there was absolutely no sign after seven weeks. No one
could tell, not even him. Incidentally, that's going fantastically well. We're moving in together.*

MARIE

Remember Marie, the happy teacher with the unhappy face?
She's now smiling on the inside *and* the outside.

*I'm fifty-eight years old, and I didn't come to this decision
lightly. I've been thinking about getting cosmetic surgery for
twenty years. What took me so long to decide? I believe it
was because I came of age in the late sixties and early seventies. Feminism was in; being natural was in. I've always
prided myself on being a natural person. I don't wear a lot
of makeup. I thought, "Am I being really vain? Am I being
selfish and superficial?" It's not your looks; it's your personality and character that are important. That was my
greatest pull back and forth. My feminist side gave me this
tug, and it took me a long time to get over that.*

*I finally got to the stage where I thought, "No, unfortunately, there is ageism in our society. You do need to look
young and fit and healthy." I look after myself. I exercise, I eat
right, I run half marathons. I've got lots of energy, but I'd look
at my aging face and think, "Oh, my God, this isn't good!"*

My face is something that I really don't have a lot of control over. It's my genes. I've got a British background, and they tend not to have the greatest skin in the world. And my mother is extremely wrinkled and old-looking. Then I thought, "It'll make me feel better to do it."

At first I worried about my eyes. I'd developed that droopy, tired look. I got used to it, got on with life, and didn't think about it anymore. The next thing that started to bother me was my neck. I'd started wearing turtlenecks and stuff, because, suddenly, the neck area was kind of sagging down. I don't know—something happens to you. All of a sudden, you look in the mirror and think, "Oh my gosh, where did that come from?"

I'm an optimist. I always feel that if something's wrong, there's a solution. Now, you have no control over some things in life, so you've got to let those things go, but this is something that you can do.

And so then, after literally twenty years of reading everything I could, I thought to myself, "Okay, I can do this as long as I find the best surgeon." I narrowed it down to seven or eight. Dr. Adamson's name came up from different medical sources. I knew a nurse who had done some training with him. A friend of my sister, who was also in the medical profession, had heard of him.

I went to see him and said, "Look, I don't even care if I look younger, I just want to look fresher and more alive. I don't care if you're taking ten years off or five years off or two years off."

What will my friends think? I'm still concerned about that. I haven't really told friends; I've only told my immediate family.

But I still wasn't sure. I hadn't even told my husband about this. I was going to tell him, of course, but I didn't want him to see me all bandaged and bruised. We don't have kids, and we kind of dote on each other. I thought I'd go to a hotel for five or six days after and just stay out of sight.

And when I finally told my husband, he practically had a heart attack thinking about it. We've always said to one another that if there's something one of us feels really strongly about, the other will support it. So, we talked about it for a few hours, and he said, "Okay, if you really want this, we'll go for it." He wouldn't contribute a penny to it because he felt if anything happened to me he could never forgive himself. So that was fine, you know. So that's the way we did it.

The staff told me I was going to need someone with me in the days after surgery, if just for emotional support. I was thinking I'd get my mother and my sister. Then the doctor told me I really should have my husband with me, and I thought, "Oh, I don't want to get him involved. He's going to be so worried."

So they encouraged me to get my husband involved, and that was the best thing I did—absolutely. He came down and met everybody there, and he felt much more comfortable with the whole thing. He was the best support

I could have imagined. I mean, he was tending to my stitches, and, you know, you do need somebody who's not afraid. My mother and my sister, in retrospect, would have been dreadful, because there are stitches and other things you have to do.

But I just felt positive. Dr. Adamson was the only surgeon I talked to, which is the absolute wrong thing to do. You're supposed to see a minimum of three. Some people see thirty, I've read. The person I read about who saw thirty said that she thought she'd made a mistake, which I thought was kind of interesting.

My instincts were that this was the thing to do and this was the person to do it. The staff was amazing, and I knew I was going to get great care. Like, during the surgery, there was Dr. Adamson, Dr. Litner, a surgical nurse, and an anesthesiologist, all for me.

The anesthesia was my biggest concern, but I thought that the risks were really minimized here. I just went with them, and I'm glad I did it.

I wouldn't have gone into this unless I had been totally healthy, because I think that's key. Dr. Adamson said most of the patients that come to him are fit and healthy. That was really important to me. There was a time when I ran three times a week for an hour, but now I'm more into walking. I still do weights and aerobics two or three times a week. I love kayaking and cross-country skiing. I'm very much an outdoorsy kind of person. I exercise a minimum of five times an week for an hour.

So I was pretty fit, and I'm still fit. And I really trained at this, almost like training for a marathon. My nutrition was great; I even cut out caffeine. You don't have to do that, but they give you huge lists of things that you've got to avoid, even certain vitamins, because they're blood-thinners. So I think I was a really good patient. I really tried hard, and I thought that there are people in Hollywood whose lifestyles aren't that great, and they get it done and are fine.

My husband was beside himself the day of the surgery. He drove me nuts. I think he called about six times. And then when I was out of it, he came up to make sure I was all right. I was aware, and I waved at him and smiled at him and said "Hi." He was thrilled with that, so that was good.

The night of the surgery wasn't the greatest. I wasn't at my best then, but I came back really well.

I had very little pain. I was uncomfortable the night of the surgery, but I think that was because I'd been under all day, so I wasn't really tired and I had these compression things on my legs for blood clots. I had a blood pressure monitor going. So I wanted to sleep, but couldn't really sleep because all these things were going on. I had to go to the bathroom, and everything had to be taken off. I felt sorry for the night nurse.

I came home. Going to a hotel would have been a disaster for me. I looked dreadful. The first few days were bad. I couldn't look in the mirror.

My husband was okay with it, but not my sister. I had the surgery on a Tuesday, and she was here on Wednesday. I had even told my mother to keep her away because she was going to have a fit when she saw me. And she did. She said, "Are you going to stay like that?" I was all swollen and deformed, so I said, "Yeah, I'm going to stay like this!"

After a week, I still had quite a bit of swelling, but my bruising was minimal. I wasn't looking too bad. If you'd met me on the street, you wouldn't have thought that I looked strange.

After two weeks, I was out shopping, doing a few little things. I didn't see anybody close, other than my family. I didn't see any friends or anything, but I'd say I was pretty good.

The improvement was stunning. Even my husband, who thought I hadn't needed it, said, "You look fabulous."

I'll be seeing my close friends in the next week or so. I've had my hair cut a little bit. I also have new glasses. They might notice something's a little different. I think I'll be able to get away with it. At some point, I might tell people, but right now, I don't want to.

Although I haven't seen friends yet, I have seen neighbors. One told me I looked good and asked if I had lost weight. And I said, "I don't think so. Maybe a couple of pounds," because I actually had lost a couple of pounds with the surgery; you don't eat for a couple of days. Another day, I was walking down the street, and a neighbor I hadn't seen for a while said to me, "I thought you were a teenager."

I think it was one of the best decisions I've made. I'd do it again in a heartbeat.

For Marta and Mary, it was simply about looking like themselves—only better.

MARTA

I don't look like a china doll or a Barbie but have retained my character expressions. I still look like me but fifteen years younger. No one has asked me if I had something done to my face, but everyone, without exception, has told me how great I look.

The true test came when I went to my cosmetician, whom I've been seeing every month for the last fourteen years. When I arrived for my appointment three weeks after surgery, she stared at me, then burst out, "You look so f——ing good. I'm going to die with envy."

MARY

I frequently see aging movie stars interviewed on TV who have obviously had face-lifts. Often the results are so artificial that it's hard to recognize them. I was afraid of ending up with that stretched, startled-eye appearance.

I had nothing to fear. The best thing about my facial surgery is how natural I look. Less than four weeks after my surgery, I hosted my extended family of twenty people at our annual Christmas dinner. Everyone commented on how great I looked. Several suggested that it must be my new hairdo (I had combed my hair over my ears to cover the fresh scars). My mother-in-law stated that wearing my glasses made me look younger (I wore these to hide the last bit of puffiness around my eyes). Some of my relatives remarked that it must be my recent retirement that was responsible for my well-rested, fresh appearance.

Having facial surgery hasn't made me look like a thirty-year-old again. But, wherever I go, whatever I'm wearing, no matter how little makeup I have on my face, I feel like a very well-preserved sixty-plus woman who always looks her best and is aging amazingly well. I have a new confidence in my appearance and a new bounce in my step.

JULIA

After her face-lift in 2002, Julia wrote a poem to express how she felt.

It's faces that you sculpt.
Expressive
Living, loving, hoping, fearing
No two alike.
But your children
Will never find them
On a museum shelf.
No dead clay or marble
Takes your strokes.
Your fingers and eyes work their magic
On living bone and blood and skin
Correcting nature's careless touch
Or softening and erasing
The traces of time's passage.

Despite the beauty of your work
No Pygmalion fears
Haunt your dreams.
For all your creations live
Re-animated with a sigh
Anonymously altered
To return to their lives and lovers.

You never even sign your work.

CHAPTER TWELVE

Besides being an ornament to the face,
a breathing apparatus, or a convenient
handle by which to grasp an impudent fellow,
(the nose) is an important index to its owner's
character.

– George Jabet, Notes on Noses

THE NOSE

Tell me about your nose. What does it look like? How is it shaped?

If you like your nose—if you're content with the appendage hanging from the front of your face—then you'll probably have to think for a minute about how to describe it.

If, on the other hand, I asked you to tell me about your eyes, or the eyes of the person nearest and dearest to you, you'd probably launch into an immediate and detailed description— the color, the shape, the curve of the brows, the subtle way they change with a smile or a frown.

The eyes are the first thing we notice when we look at a human face. The nose, for all its front and center presence, is barely in the picture. But there's one exception—and it's a big one.

THE PREOCCUPATION WITH YOUR NOSE

If you don't like your nose, then noses—yours and others—get top billing when it comes to looking at your face and the faces of others. And if I ask you to describe your nose, the nose you dislike, you'll be able to speak at length about it without a second's hesitation. You'll have ready opinions about noses in general. You'll be a nose expert. You might be like Susan, who, dismayed by her own nose's slight dorsal bump and droopy tip, developed a nose for noses.

"I examine just about every nose I meet," she says. "With the best noses, I try to find some telltale sign of a nose job. I've been known to approach total strangers with, 'You have a great nose,' hoping this would spur on some rhino rhetoric. I'm actually pretty good at spotting a 'done' nose."

There's an old saying: He who has a great nose thinks everybody is speaking of it. You think—no, you're absolutely *sure*—that it stands out, as H.G. Wells lamented of his own nose, "like a bit of primordial chaos."

You may be supremely self-conscious, like Kimberly, the shy nurse who tried to hide on the subway. "I was constantly aware of my nose," she says. "The only place I felt comfortable was in the privacy of my own home."

Patient Jillian, whose crooked nose got even more crooked after a competitive downhill skiing accident, reported being unhappy with it since her teens. "I felt self-conscious when people looked at me from the side as I thought my nose looked ugly," she says.

Perhaps you're like Sarah. At family events where photographs were being taken, she always rushed to get in position on the right so that the photographer wouldn't capture her "bad side."

When a patient comes in to see me about rhinoplasty, I'll say that most people don't talk about their noses very much. Most might say that John or Susie has nice-looking eyes or a great smile or nice hair, because those are the things that you notice first. They like their noses and take them for granted. But then I'll say, "I know you notice noses a lot because you're looking at noses and thinking, 'That's a nice nose. I wouldn't mind a nose like that' or 'Gosh, I wonder why she doesn't get her nose done. It looks so unattractive.'" And every one of them will tell me that this is exactly how it is.

If someone dislikes his or her nose when they're young, he or she will dislike it to the day he or she dies. It doesn't mean that he or she has to have rhinoplasty, but he or she won't grow out of it. And that's why we see ourselves doing rhinoplasties even on fifty-, sixty-, and seventy-year-olds. On the other hand, if someone comes in at the age of fifty or even younger and says he or she has only disliked his or her nose for six months or a year, that's a red flag for me. There may be something else going on in that person's life that rhinoplasty won't fix.

Rhinoplasty can make your nose smaller and narrower (or bigger and wider, for that matter). It can make a crooked nose straighter. It can remove bumps, reshape the tip, and change the angle between the nose and the upper lip. If you've ever broken your nose, if it has collided with a door, a hockey stick, or anything else, you may have problems breathing through it. Rhinoplasty can correct that too. In short, a nose job can work wonders.

But these are all physical changes. Something else also goes on with rhinoplasty patients. They can undergo emotional and psychological changes for the better. A fifty-year-old woman with an aging face problem will feel good about herself after a face-lift because her outer appearance will match her inner self. She'll look the way she feels. A rhinoplasty patient often struggles with more profound issues. The nose has great psychological, emotional, social, and symbolic importance. In their study of the psychological effects of plastic surgery, John and Marcia Goin observe, "Our literary, mythic and folkloric heritage abounds with references to it. We say that people are nosy or hard-nosed, or that they have their noses to the grindstone. We count noses, look down them, nose out competitors and win by a nose."

A lifetime of self-consciousness about a nose that somehow isn't right—that you believe causes others to look down *their* noses at you—can set off a cascade of consequences.

As a high schooler, Kimberly wanted to be a trial lawyer but, because of her nose, couldn't bear the thought of standing up and arguing a case in front of a courtroom full of people. Later, when her marriage hit the rocks, she found a way to blame it on her nose.

THE HISTORY OF NOSES

History is full of superstition, rash judgments, and pseudoscience about the nose. There was a long-standing belief that an individual's character isn't just stamped on his or her face but spelled out in the lines and contours of the appendage on the front of his or her face.

The ancients could look at a face and leap headlong into all kinds of conclusions about its owner. The Roman poet Ovid believed that "the truth of a man lies in his nose." The Romans had a thing about noses. In close combat, they aimed for the nose, letting the enemies of Rome wear their defeat on their faces.

The First Nose Job

Ours is an old profession. The first rhinoplasties were performed not decades ago, not centuries ago, but more than 2,600 years ago.

The place was India. The surgeon was Sushruta, a teacher of medicine. He was a busy guy. That's because adulterers not only got thrown out of their houses but also had their noses cut off.

Sushruta could put things right. He compiled the first step-by-step guide to rhinoplasty.

- Gather a vine leaf big enough to cover the severed piece of nose.
- Slice from the cheek a patch of living flesh equal to the size of the leaf.
- Scarify the severed piece of nose with a knife and quickly apply the cheek skin to the area.
- Insert two small pipes in the nostrils to allow breathing and to keep the graft from hanging down.
- Dust the nose with pulverized sappanwood, licorice root, and barberry to aid healing.

- Bind the severed nose piece back in place with cotton, and sprinkle it with sesame oil.
- When healing is complete, trim off the excess skin.

And, Sushruta might have added, don't cheat on your spouse.

Noses and Character

In her book *The Nose: A Profile of Sex, Beauty and Survival*, American journalist Gabrielle Glaser (the proud owner of a magnificent nose) describes how the nose was central to the eighteenth-century revival of the pseudoscience of physiognomy (judging character on the basis of appearance). Swiss theologian Johann Kaspar Lavater published essays in which he analyzed his subjects' noses, foreheads, eyes, and chins. According to Glaser, a quick glance at anyone was all Lavater needed to understand a person's morality, intelligence, and religiosity.

Lavater's strange preoccupation caught on. Faces, and particularly noses, were the key to character. It boiled down to this: Fine features meant goodness, while coarse features were bad. Such nonsense almost cost Charles Darwin his berth on HMS *Beagle*, the ship of discovery that carried him to the Galapagos Islands, where his studies of the unique animal life led to the theory of evolution. Captain Robert FitzRoy didn't want Darwin on board as the ship's naturalist because of his bulbous nose. "He was an ardent disciple of Lavater and was convinced he could judge a man's character by the outline of his features," Darwin wrote, "and he doubted whether anyone with my nose could possess sufficient energy and determination for the voyage." FitzRoy relented, and Darwin wrote,

"I think he was afterwards well-satisfied that my nose had spoken falsely."

Napoleon famously said that an army marches on its stomach, but he believed the success of that army could be found higher on the body—in the noses of his officers. He equated big noses with big brains. "When I want any good head-work done I choose a man . . . with a long nose," he wrote.

The writing of Honoré de Balzac, a nineteenth-century master of literary realism, is full of plotlines that hinge on the size and shape of his characters' noses. Many of his novels and short stories are collected within *La Comédie Humaine*. It contains no fewer than 400 references to noses. The "realism" of his descriptions leaves room for doubt.

In *The Vicar of Tours*, Mlle. Gamard, an unhappy woman, runs a boarding house for priests and has no friends. Why? The answer was as plain as the nose on her face. "Her aquiline nose was of all her facial characteristics the one that did most to express the despotism of her ideas, just as the flattened angle of her forehead betrayed the narrowness of her mind."

Another Frenchman, Edmond Rostand, built a classic play, *Cyrano de Bergerac*, around a nose. "A great nose indicates a great man," said Cyrano, "genial, courteous, intellectual, virile [and] courageous."

Classification of Noses

It wasn't just the French who put enormous stock in the nose. In 1854, across the English Channel in London, George Jabet wrote a book called *Notes on Noses* that satirized the work of Lavater and other physiognomists by arguing that the mind and the personality were inextricably linked to the size and shape of the nose.

Jabet came up with a five-part system for classifying masculine noses and thereby determining the characters of their
owners:

- One: The Roman or aquiline nose revealed energy and firm-
ness in its owner, but an "absence of refinement."
- Two: Refinement of character was to be found in the Greek
or straight nose. Possessors of such noses were lovers of the
fine arts. In Jabet's classification system, this nose gets four
stars. "It is the highest and most beautiful form the organ
can assume."
- Three: The cogitative nose, which gradually widens from
below the bridge, revealed a big brain. Here, Jabet cautions
his readers to always judge noses not just in profile but from
the front as well, lest they miss the cogitative nose.
- Four: The Jewish or hawk nose (thin and sharp) was a sure
sign of shrewdness and insight "and facility of turning that
insight into profitable account."
- Five: The snub and celestial noses were fine, even desirable
in women, but in men, it revealed "natural weakness, a
mean disagreeable disposition, petty insolence," and many
other appalling character traits.

Jabet applied his tongue-in-cheek theory of noses worldwide,
with politically incorrect conclusions. Every country, he wrote,
has a national nose. The most advanced countries are noted for
their Greek noses; the lesser for their snubs. Here, non–Anglo
Saxons got the short end of the stick.

Viewed now, it's surprising how people embraced such
beliefs. But they did. "A gentleman with a pug nose," wrote
Edgar Allan Poe, "is a contradiction in terms."

Michelangelo's Flat Nose

He painted the ceiling of the Sistine Chapel lying on his back and breathing through his mouth. Michelangelo's nose was a singularly unlovely sight, squashed so flat against his face that, in the words of one historian, "his forehead almost overhung [it]."

The great Renaissance artist fell victim to a sucker punch that didn't just break his nose but pulverized it. And it happened in church.

Michelangelo, just a boy at the time and learning his craft in Florence, had the habit of rubbing people the wrong way. He was considered the up-and-coming new star—and he knew it. He irritated other artists by making fun of their work. One day, he went too far. He and fellow artist Pietro Torrigiano, three years his senior, were in the Brancacci chapel of the Carmine church to study what was even then a Florentine masterpiece, the Masaccio frescoes. "One day in particular when he was bothering me, I became much more irritated than usual and, clenching my fist, I dealt him such a blow on the nose that I felt the bone and the cartilage crumble under my fist as if they had been made of crisp wafer," Torrigiano later told a friend. "He'll go with my mark on him to his dying day," Torrigiano added.

And he did. Michelangelo went on to flat-nosed greatness in Florence and Rome. Torrigiano fled to "barbarian" Britain, where he fell in with another pugnacious fellow, King Henry VIII.

Tycho's Golden Nose

Danish astronomer Tycho Brahe, who lived in the late sixteenth century, was brilliant but hot-headed and eccentric. He had a castle and a pet moose. (The moose later got drunk on beer, fell down a staircase, and died.)

Brahe and Danish nobleman Manderup Parsbjerg, in their cups at an engagement party, got into an argument. More than two weeks later, the quarrel resumed, this time with rapiers. Parsbjerg proved to be the better swordsman. He neatly sliced off most of Brahe's nose.

Brahe reappeared weeks later with an artificial nose made from an alloy of gold and silver. He carried a small box of paste that he used to hold his golden nose in place.

NOSES AND SEX

So the nose carries with it a lot of excess baggage. No wonder it's one of the most psychologically loaded of all the body parts. And it's not just about intelligence and personality. It's also about something far more primal: sex. The eyes may be the windows of the soul, but the nose is the face's true sexy beast.

In their book on the psychological effects of plastic surgery, John and Marcia Goin (one a surgeon, the other a psychiatrist) rank the nose with the breast and the penis as the most important organs in terms of psychology and sex. The nose, it's argued, is a secondary sex organ. Consider this: The male nose is one of only two protruding midline anatomical structures. It undergoes a growth spurt at adolescence, and it emits a sticky mucous substance. Sound familiar? The nose and the penis have much in common.

But the comparisons don't stop with males. In breathing, the nose is primarily receptive—like female genitalia. It's a cavernous structure that sometimes bleeds. Beyond that, it sometimes becomes stuffy after sex, causing so-called honeymoon rhinitis.

Over the centuries, doctors have equated the nose, fixations with the nose, and problems with the nose (including runny noses) with various kinds of sexual dysfunction. Glaser tells of German doctor Wilhelm Fliess, a late nineteenth-century ear, nose, and throat specialist who argued that the nose has its own form of menstrual cycle. Fliess claimed that "genital spots" in the nose grew swollen with "sexual substances" once a month. This, he believed, caused a kind of sexual hysteria. His treatment involved a snort of cocaine. If that didn't work, he followed up with the surgical removal of part of the nasal bone. The great Viennese psychoanalyst Sigmund Freud befriended Fliess, shared cocaine with him for his own stuffy nose, and even referred one of his patients to Fleiss for this surgery. It went badly, and the patient almost died. Such was the preoccupation with the nose. Others blamed it for all kinds of physical, emotional, and mental problems, including retardation. Children with stuffy noses and children who breathed through their mouths were judged as "slow" and, worse, more likely to masturbate.

The nose has always been symbolically sexual, a genital equivalent, say the Goins. But the sexual connection isn't just symbolic. Way in the back of the nose sits the tiny vomeronasal organ, which is mainly used to detect pheromones, chemical substances that humans and other animals produce to stimulate behavioral responses in others of the same species, including powerful sexual signals. When couples talk about having "good chemistry," they may not know it, but they're most likely responding to each other's pheromones. In histology, the science of organic tissues, the mucous membranes of the nose closely resemble erectile tissue in the male genitalia. Viewed this way, the nose and the penis are first cousins.

It's no wonder, then, that psychiatrists' couches are full of people blaming sexual problems on their noses. It's called displacement. For plastic surgeons, initial meetings with prospective rhinoplasty patients are critically important. For example, if someone in middle age has only just started disliking his or her nose, this can be a huge red flag for the plastic surgeon. It may not be the nose he or she hates. It may be something else, something connected with sex, a failed relationship, a concern about sexual performance, or even a concern about sexual identity. The study of the nose abounds with a bizarre combination of fact and fiction. Emotional and sexual problems often seem like one and the same. But it's possible to get carried away in making the connection.

Half a century ago, professors at an American university looked for a link between garden-variety nasal problems, such as stuffiness and sneezing, and depression and anxiety. Their case studies, as Glaser reports, bore telling titles. One was called "Chronic Disease of the Sinuses and Vasomotor Rhinitis in an Anxious, Dissatisfied, Frustrated, Resentful Woman who Based her Security on her 'Good Looks' and 'Sexual Assets', and Who Feared She Was Losing Both." Another was titled "Nasal Obstruction in an Insecure, Dependent, Ambitious, Lachrymose Man." You get the idea. The authors, Glaser says, claimed there were "clear links between humiliation, rejection, anxiety, and dejection to everything from runny noses to sinus disease."

PSYCHOLOGY AND NOSES

Can anxiety announce itself in the nose? Yes. Is the nose a secondary sexual organ, as the Goins say? I believe so. But are sneezing and stuffiness signs of frustration and resentment? Of course not. These are usually the sign of allergies or a cold.

Can seeking to change the size and shape of your nose be seen as a denial of your ethnicity? Historically, yes, and sometimes for good reasons—reasons of self-preservation. During the Third Reich, Germany barred citizenship to all but those of Aryan ancestry. That ruled out Jews. It was an early step in the anti-Semitic measures that led to the Holocaust. Many German Jews had rhinoplasties to hide their ethnicity and protect their jobs and, ultimately, their lives.

The Goins say the desire for rhinoplasty can also be psychologically linked to relationships within families. Patients who, for whatever reason, harbor animosity toward a parent or grandparent sometimes seek to rid themselves of a characteristic family nose.

THE PROCESS OF RHINOPLASTY

So the nose bears a huge load of emotional and psychological baggage for its owner. The goal of rhinoplasty is to make the nose blend in. It may be the most prominent feature on the face, but it shouldn't be distracting. It's all about first impressions—what you see when you first set eyes on someone. It takes one-sixth of a second to scan a face. In that fleeting moment, the gaze shouldn't stop at the nose but go straight to the eyes. That means creating a nose that looks balanced, proportional, and feminine or masculine, as the case may be—a nose that people just don't notice.

That makes the nose tricky and delicate terrain for the plastic surgeon. It's always approached with great caution. Rhinoplastic surgery involves dozens of basic steps, each affecting all the others. Imagine a watch that's two centimeters in diameter. Suppose that you want to make a watch that looks the same, but 18 millimeters in diameter. Every little wheel in that entire watch has to be changed and fitted appropriately. That's what rhinoplasty is like. You're dealing with complex anatomical structures.

First, the septum (the midline wall) usually has to be straightened. Most of us are asymmetrical to varying degrees, up to and including our noses. One study showed 97 percent of patients undergoing rhinoplasty had asymmetrical faces.

Then there's the tip of the nose. It may be too long or too short. Changing that can involve cutting and shortening the cartilage arch, but it may also mean taking cartilage from the nose, and sometimes from the ear or even a rib, to use as struts to support the arch.

The dorsum, the bone at the bridge of the nose, may have to be reduced. A misstep here can result in a nose that looks great in profile but oddly flat when seen from the front.

When all that's done, the skin has to once again rest easily and naturally on its reshaped foundation.

For all these reasons, rhinoplasty is the most difficult cosmetic facial surgery procedure to get just right. These are the things a surgeon thinks about when assessing a prospective rhinoplasty patient. There's a lot of planning. By the time I take a scalpel to a patient's nose, I've gone over the case four times, first in the initial consultation, then in more detail in the follow-up consultation. I then plan the operation, writing down what we expect to do during surgery. The fourth time I go over the operation is the night before or the morning of surgery, when I review my plan and consider the various things I intend to do. The fifth time is the surgery itself.

CHAPTER THIRTEEN

Bah! The thing is not a nose at all, but a bit of primordial chaos clapped on to my face.

— *H.G. Wells*, author

LOLA'S RHINOPLASTY

Lola, a public health worker, is a single woman in her twenties. She's tall and slim, with the striking good looks of a fashion model. She's a happy camper—except for her nose.

CONSULTATIONS

We meet at an initial consultation and get to know each other over about an hour. I already know something about the general state of her health because she's filled out the standard health questionnaire, a requirement for every patient stepping into a doctor's office for the first time. Physically, she appears to be a good candidate for elective surgery.

I learn about her concerns with her nose. Lola tells me that she can see it tilting slightly to the left. I see the same thing, seat Lola in front of a mirror, and show her how rhinoplasty can make an improvement. We take photographs for the next meeting.

A few days later, Lola decides to go ahead. She books a planning meeting where Dr. Litner, who's doing a one-year fellowship, goes through the details of her surgery and recovery. He makes sure that she's aware of the risks, however small, of going under a general anesthetic and having this kind of operation. They agree upon a surgery date.

PREPARATIONS

"The getting ready" recommendations Lola received are straightforward. She stocks up on soft foods, liquids, and bendable drinking straws. She arranges for her mother to take her home after surgery and stay with her overnight. She also follows the hard-and-fast rules. She avoids pills containing aspirin (e.g., Aspirin, Advil, Bufferin, 222s, Triaminic tablets) for two weeks prior to surgery, as they're blood thinners and may cause excess bleeding during surgery. She also avoids herbal remedies, including echinacea, garlic, ginseng, green tea, and chamomile tea, as they're also blood thinners.

SURGERY

Lola's rhinoplasty, done under general anesthetic, takes one hour and forty minutes. It begins with an incision beneath the tip of the nose and is carried along to the inside of each nostril. The skin of the nose is then freed up from the underlying tissue and elevated. Now the inside of the nose is exposed.

The first step is to remove some cartilage from the midline of the nose. Small cuts are made in the crura, a number of arch-shaped segments that form a dome-like structure and give the tip of the nose its shape. The crura are then sculpted into their new position and sewn back together. Some of the removed cartilage is reshaped and put back in beneath the tip and along the sides to support the "new" nose.

We move on to the bridge of the nose. It has to be lowered slightly. It's shaved down slightly with an instrument similar to a file. Small cuts are made in the bone with a few taps on a chisel-like instrument called an osteotome. This breaks the nose, enabling me to reshape the bridge. The skin is re-draped on the new frame, and the incisions are closed.

A small cast is placed on the nose, and plastic splints are inserted in the nostrils. A small amount of gauze is placed at the nostril openings.

AFTER SURGERY

The next day, Lola looks puffy, swollen, and bruised. She also has two black eyes. Lola's nose feels blocked up, as the tissues are swollen and the splints are still in place. It's no walk-in-the-park day. Lola feels miserable. "The things I do for beauty," she says.

The little bit of gauze comes out the day after surgery. Three days later, we snip and remove the external sutures that have been holding the nose together. Internal sutures remain, but they'll dissolve on their own.

The cast comes off in eight days, and so do the splints that have been placed inside the nostrils. By then, Lola is feeling much better. Most of the swelling and bruising disappears. Lola is given a list of postoperative instructions to follow.

POSTOPERATIVE INSTRUCTIONS

Do . . .	Do not . . .
– Keep a cold washcloth or gauze over your eyes and upper cheeks as much as possible for the first thirty-six hours after surgery. – Drink plenty of fluids. Your throat will be dry. – Keep your mouth open if you have to sneeze. – Use a humidifier. – Keep a stiff upper lip—literally. Don't move the upper lip too much in the week after surgery. – Be careful around rambunctious children or spouses who move around in bed a lot. Your nose isn't in any condition to be accidentally smacked right now. – Use cotton swabs and hydrogen peroxide to gently clean your nostrils and visible stitches.	– Go overboard on talking, smiling, and vigorous tooth brushing. Brush gently (or with your finger). – Eat anything that's hard to chew or that may upset your stomach. – Wear your glasses for six weeks after surgery. They could play havoc with the healing of the nasal bones. If you absolutely need your glasses, we can show you a way to support them on your face but not on your nose. – Do any vigorous exercise or lift anything heavier than a bag of potatoes. – Sniff or blow your nose for ten days after surgery. This will be bothersome. – Use nose drops.

– Climb the pain-medication ladder. If you need a pain reliever, try Tylenol (but no aspirin-based medications). If that doesn't work, use your prescription pain medication (we'll give you the prescription).	– Go anywhere near a hot tub for three weeks. – Drive for a week. – Do aerobic activities or workouts for two to three weeks. – Play contact sports for six weeks.

When can she resume her life? For some activities, such as shampooing, it's just a day or two as long as the nose is kept dry. She can have a bath right away, even a shower if the water isn't too hot. Smoking and drinking can be resumed in two weeks, though many smokers use their facial plastic surgery as an opportune time to stop smoking for good. Most patients may resume normal professional and social activities after two weeks.

It'll take about six weeks until Lola's nose feels back to normal. It will continue to refine, and there can be residual numbness in the tip for up to a year. A month after surgery, she takes a holiday in Mexico.

CHAPTER FOURTEEN

*There is nothing so difficult to marry
as a large nose.*

—*Oscar Wilde,* An Ideal Husband

BRAD AND ARPI—THE NOSE DIARIES

Rhinoplasty is like painting or sculpting in a patient's tissues. The last day I do one—and I will have done thousands of them—I know that it will still be a challenge and I'll still be trying to do things better.

If you've decided to have rhinoplasty, you'll want to know what will happen and how you'll feel before and after. You'll also want tips on what to do and what to avoid as you prepare for and recover from your big journey. Allow me to introduce you to Brad and Arpi, two of my rhinoplasty patients who provided detailed accounts of their experiences—before, during, and after surgery.

BRAD

Brad, a young computer programmer, says that he'd had a good nose until puberty and then it became crooked. That's typical.

Often people say that a bump grew in their teens and they feel it was due to an accident. They must have broken it. It's usually just congenital. It's the nature of the nose.

People who consult me about their noses are usually specific about the problem. They don't like the bump or the droopy tip or the length. They usually say that they want it smaller. Not Brad. Brad was even more specific: He wanted his nose reduced by 10 percent. Here is Brad's story. In his own words, it's "an almost perfectly normal boy's journal."

-1-

Big and Crooked

"Hey! What the heck. My nose doesn't look straight. Let's see. No. No. It definitely has a curve in it. Hmm. It can't be that noticeable, though. I mean, I just saw it now."

I'm sixteen years old, looking in the mirror and seeing that my teenage growth spurt isn't exactly treating me very fairly. Isn't it bad enough that I'm skinny as a rail and have just started on tetracycline for my acne? Now I have to contend with a nose that's clearly getting too big—and crooked. Great! Just fantastic! But still, I'm resilient. I have a good group of friends. I'm smart and funny, and I know very well that, physically speaking, nobody's perfect. Besides, I'm still a growing teenager. Eventually I'll become a good-looking adult. Right? Wrong!

At school, a classmate turns to me and says, "What happened to your nose? It's all . . . " [he grabs his own nose and pretends to twist it out of shape while making a groaning noise]. *I quickly came up with a lie. I tell him I broke it when*

I was younger and can't get it fixed until I stop growing. He buys the lie and never mentions my nose again. But the thing is, I buy it too. I realize that the flaws in my face (which I'd barely noticed in the past) are more obvious than I thought— and are perhaps even becoming worse. I tell myself that someday I'll be getting these flaws corrected. There's no way I'm going to have to deal with this for the rest of my life.

-2-

I Got Shafted!

I'm seventeen and make my first appointment with a local cosmetic surgeon. I can't afford any procedures but am interested in learning more about what can be done and how much it will cost. Yeah, it's going to be expensive, but one day . . . I hope.

By the time I'm twenty, I'm six feet tall and weigh just 130 pounds. Beyond that, I still have major acne problems. Add to that a long nose that veers off to the left as if it had been broken in a fight, and you get the picture. What the heck happened to genetics? The rest of my family is picture-perfect. I got shafted!

Girlfriends are few and far between. But one day, I strike gold—or so I think. She's a tall, traffic-stopping blonde with a Barbie doll figure. And she wants me! I have to say the relationship is purely physical. We aren't the best match, and, frankly, she's driving me into the poorhouse. Did I mention that she's an exotic dancer? I believe now that my poor body image kept me hanging onto the relationship far longer than I should have. After all, she was genuinely physically attracted to me, and girls like her don't normally date guys like me.

Fortunately, the relationship ends after a couple of years. So here I am, single again, mid-twenties, skinny as a rail, acne, blah, blah, blah. We've heard it all before. I decide to concentrate on improving my self-image, saving some money, accomplishing some goals, lifting some weights and, I hope, growing out of my acne.

-3-

Now It's My Chin

With the age of thirty quickly approaching, I'm feeling better about myself in general. I'd definitely excelled in some areas of my life and had a lot to be proud of. But I'm watching friends get married and realizing that being single really stinks. I still get the occasional zit, but nothing I can't contend with. I'm a little heavier but not exactly where I want to be in that department. As for my nose, well, it's still undeniably large and crooked. If that isn't enough, I now begin to notice something else—my chin. I guess because I wear a goatee and rarely see myself well from the side, I never realized how underdeveloped my chin is. I had noticed it before but never fully realized the impact it had on my overall appearance. In fact, I'm now sure my chin is only amplifying the issues with my nose. What next?

I enjoy watching educational channels on TV. I see a show on human attraction and realize how some women must feel, being bombarded with images of impossible-to-achieve female figures. I'm sitting here watching how I'm basically the opposite of what biologically attracts a woman to a man—muscle development, left-to-right symmetry, strong jawline. Interesting as these shows are, I find them damaging to my body image and self-esteem. I'm the most self-conscious about my appearance that I've ever been.

I research rhinoplasty and chin augmentation on the Internet. I learn that a crooked nose is one of the most difficult things to fix and can rarely be corrected 100 percent.

I'm thinking about this as my family's big summer barbeque approaches. Children are present, young eight- to ten-year-olds who can be painfully truthful. One of them tells me, pointedly, that my nose looks like a witch's nose—not just any witch's nose, but the nose of the witch in the new Harry Potter movie. That's it! I decide then and there that I will get surgery as soon as possible.

-4-

Taking the Plunge

It's now fall. I start saving money for the surgery. I hope to have enough in about a year—maybe even as early as next spring. I decide to keep my goatee and current hairstyle until after the surgery. Then I'll change everything and help draw attention away from the major changes in my face.

Spring comes and I'm not yet ready. The surgery must wait until fall.

It's midsummer. I schedule appointments with two cosmetic surgeons. The first one is very nice and so is his staff. He tells me everything I want to hear about the surgery, the procedures, and the outcome. I'm given some forms for blood work and told to schedule an appointment for surgery when I'm ready.

My next appointment is with Dr. Adamson. He goes into greater detail and cautions me that the procedure to straighten my nose is difficult to get perfect. Improvement must be the goal, not perfection. This is something I already know from my research, but I appreciate hearing it from him. He goes over the additional consultations, tests, and photographs that will be needed to paint the whole picture of my situation. This attention to detail impresses me. I schedule surgery for one month later.

Over that month, I have various appointments for consultations, photographs, and tests to prepare for the operation. I arrange to stay at a friend's house during the time after surgery. I'm surprisingly calm as the day of surgery approaches, but I've been quite busy.

-5-

The Big Day

On surgery day, I get up, shower, and jump in a cab for the clinic, perhaps a little nervous, but not freaking out. I arrive and change into a gown, and Dr. Adamson comes in to prepare me. He marks the location for my chin implant and asks if I have any questions. This is my last chance to run for the door, but that's the last thing I want to do. I'm excited about having this lifelong goal achieved.

I enter the operating room and lie on the table. The anesthetist starts a drip, and I fall unconscious in mid-conversation.

The next thing I know, I'm waking up and feeling pretty good, all things considered. With each passing minute, I become more alert. I peek in a mirror, expecting to look bad and am surprised. There's just a small cast on my nose and a bandage around my chin. I have no problem with this at all. And I can tell, even with the cast on, that there are huge changes in my nose.

-6-

An Awkward Week

My friend picks me up, and we go back to his place. I try to relax. If there was any negative time from my experience, it's here. His apartment is small, his sofa bed is uncomfortable, and his cat is annoying. I feel like an intruder and cut short my stay. My father comes to pick me up.

The first week after surgery is the most awkward. Trying to sleep in an elevated position is difficult but necessary. I sleep in a reclining chair. Luckily, I heal quickly. Bruising, while bad for a day or two, has diminished rapidly. There's very little pain. The oddest part was a complete lack of feeling in my chin and lower lip because of the implant. I knew that feeling would be lost temporarily but hadn't fully realized that it could take weeks to return.

The stitches come out a week or so after surgery. This is relatively painless—except for the stitches inside my nostrils. Ouch! The cast comes off my nose. The change is dramatic. I'm very excited about just how much straighter my nose now is. In fact, I'd have to say it was considerably better than I was expecting.

I'm back in my own bed now, but with the pillows arranged in such a manner that I remain on my back with my head slightly elevated. If my head gets too low, I find that I wake up with a fair bit of swelling in my face. Some sensation returns to my chin area, reassuring me that everything will be fine. The most difficult thing is eating with no feeling in my lower lip.

-7-

My New Look

As the weeks go by, the swelling subsides and feeling slowly but surely returns to my lip. I settle into my new appearance so rapidly that I have to refer to photographs to understand the incredible difference from before.

I change my hairstyle, modernizing it a little. I shave off my goatee. Those who know about the surgery are extremely impressed. Those who don't often comment about improvements in my appearance but are unable to tell what exactly has been improved. Usually, they think it's my hair. Female friends and family are the most observant. Men might say, "Hey, you're looking good these days." Women say, "There's something really different, but I don't know exactly what. Did you have a beard before? Maybe it's your hair."

So here I am, thirty years old, with a fantastic life going for myself—and of course a much better profile and a nearly perfect nose. Now if only I could get my lazy butt to the gym!

Her broad, flat nose, with nostrils expanded into oval cavities, breathed the fires of hell, and resembled the beak of some evil bird of prey.

– *Honoré de Balzac,* novelist and playwright

ARPI

We all shrink as we get older. It usually begins in our thirties, a little earlier than you'd expect. With advancing age, spinal tissue slowly compresses. The body seems to draw in upon itself. One part that never gets smaller is the nose. That's what Arpi discovered, and here is her story.

Once a woman tells you her age, she'll tell you anything. So here goes. I'm fifty-four—kind of late in the game for a nose job.

I have a degree in languages from the University of Toronto, and I taught high school French. Then I switched careers. I did industrial sales for five years, marketing, real estate. I reinvented myself several times job-wise because I'd stop working to raise my two daughters, and then I'd go back, depending on what their needs were. Certain periods of time were very crucial when they needed their mom around.

My older daughter is thirty, and my younger one is twenty-six. My older daughter was married in 2002 and my younger one three years later. So I'm done raising kids, and I have to say the empty nest is fabulous. I don't know why everybody complains about an empty nest. I really enjoy the quiet. It gives me time to catch up on my reading, and I've started doing more volunteer work because I've got more time.

I've got an interesting ethnic background. I'm of Armenian parentage, born in Israel and educated in a French Catholic school. We came to Canada in 1965. In the 1960s, I was involved in protests and sit-ins and all that kind of stuff. I was a late developer, like 100 pounds— skinny, you might say. I could eat everything. That was my genetic predisposition through my father's side. When I look back at the pictures, my nose wasn't prominent because it wasn't crooked, and it wasn't huge because my eyes were large and so were my cheekbones. My bone structure was fine so that the face could carry the nose without giving me any angst. I never had any problems at that stage.

As I got into my thirties, I started noticing that my nose seemed to be getting bigger while the rest of the face was shrinking. I never felt insecure or bothered because I've always gotten positive feedback from those around me.

My husband always tells me I'm beautiful, and when I told him I wanted to get my nose done, he told me I was nuts. He said, "Why? You're beautiful!" So he never saw it.

And the other reason I'd never had the operation done until now was that it was just never a priority for me. My priorities were getting my degree, then having a happy, healthy family. It seemed like kind of a frivolous thing to do.

I don't know if it was gravity or not, but the tip was leaning down and it looked like it had shifted to one side.

The tip was quite bulbous, and it bothered the heck out of me. I'm quite keen on proportion and I like beautiful things, and, as far as I was concerned, the rest of my face met my criteria of what beautiful is—but the nose didn't at this point.

My youngest daughter was about to be married, and I thought, "I'm not going to be hiding from the camera, and I'm not going to be telling the photographer, 'Don't take profiles, just frontals, no profiles.'" I didn't like feeling like that, and that made me feel defensive, as if I were apologizing and protecting something. I thought, "Why am I wasting all this mental energy on something that shouldn't be so important?"

I told my husband that it was really starting to bother me. He asked, "Why at this stage? You've lived with it all your life, why now?"

I said, "I don't know, but right now, at this time in my life, it's really bothering me." The minute I said it was really bothering me, he supported my decision to go ahead.

I did quite a bit of research on the Internet, and that's how I discovered Dr. Adamson. I did a thorough background check on him. Probably the only thing I couldn't figure out was what he'd had for breakfast that day.

I learned what the surgery entailed because I thought that if something went wrong—God forbid—and I ended up dying on the surgical table, I thought that would be really stupid. If I were going to die, there had better be a better reason than because of a stupid nose, right?

I went to Dr. Adamson and I didn't say to him, "Give me some movie star's nose." I told him that, at the end of it, after I went down under the knife, I wanted to make sure that it was still me I saw. I didn't want to see somebody else, or somebody else's nose on my face. I wanted it to still be my nose.

I told him to give me a nose that would be in proportion to my face, and he said, "Those are the only kind I do." And that's exactly what he gave me. I feel like I should have been born with this nose instead of the one I had.

And what's funny is that he told me, "Once you have your nose done, people won't know." He said, "They won't see any difference in you."

I had a thorough physical checkup beforehand, including my heart because I used to have a bit of arrhythmia. My family doctor told me not to worry, that I was an excellent candidate for surgery.

As for the surgery itself, I wasn't miserable. It was more discomfort than pain. I wasn't able to open my mouth, so I was drinking through a straw. They gave me Tylenol 3s, and I rarely take any medication, so after taking one of those pills, I was out of it.

I had been under the anesthesia a bit more than three hours, so I was drinking lots of liquids to flush the whole thing out of my system. I'd say the reason I didn't have such a bad aftereffect was that I did a lot of prep work beforehand. Mentally, I was ready to see my face all really beaten up.

On days two and three, I swelled up something terrible. I was black and blue all the way down my neck.

After the third day, the swelling went down. My eyes opened up, and the black and blue was turning into green and yellow. I worried that, because I'm older, I might be left with sagging skin because of all that bloating and bruising. Dr. Adamson assured me that this wasn't going to happen, and it didn't. After five months, it's fabulous. There's still a little swelling at the tip of my nose, but that's coming down.

This has been very positive for me. I was surprised at how positive. People come up to me and, when they haven't seen me, they say, "Oh, did you just get back from vacation?" They don't even notice that it's the nose. Or they say, "Have you had your eyes done?" because it's made my eyes pop out more, whereas before the focus was on my nose, dragging down my face.

When you look at a face, the nose is the great prominent feature, but you really don't want it to be the first thing you notice; you want the eyes to be the first thing you see when you look at someone. But I also think that it's not so much for the people around you—it's about you and about how you see yourself. I think that's what it's all about.

A couple of people have come up to me and said, "Arpi, did you have your nose done?" These are the perceptive people. I tell them I did. It's not something I hide or am ashamed of. Au contraire—I tell everybody about it.

Even though my husband has always told me I was beautiful and all that kind of stuff, the other day we were relaxing and he was looking at me in profile and said, "You know what? There is a difference."

And I said, "I told you, but you never saw it until I pointed it out to you."

The wedding pictures came back, and they look great. I'm thrilled with my results.

CHAPTER FIFTEEN

Lightly was her slender nose
Tip-tilted like the petal of a flower

— *Alfred*, Lord Tennyson, poet

DIARIES OF MAGNIFICENT NOSES

Rhinoplasty surgery—from the initial tiny incision beneath the tip of the nose to the last delicate suture—usually takes about two to three hours (depending on the complexity). But the patient's journey through rhinoplasty takes much longer. It can be difficult and fraught with anxiety. It usually begins in adolescence with that "I hate my nose" feeling. It can follow a tortuous trail with stops along the way at doubt ("I shouldn't be doing this") and fear ("What if I come out of it looking worse?"). But the final destination is, as we see from our patients' diaries, worth the trip.

SARAH

I've wanted my nose done for as long as I can remember. The desire to have it fixed would become very strong, and then I'd think that I could live with it if I could just focus on developing my self-confidence. Wanting to change my nose was surely just a reflection of a lack of self-worth, wasn't it? I managed to push the desire to the back of my mind for years, but it never went away.

Finally, when I started making enough money to allow for the possibility of considering a nose job, I started talking to friends who had had one. This "normalized" the procedure for me. It wasn't this extreme measure anymore. It was something a lot of normal people did, and they were thrilled with the results, both visually and emotionally.

I chose my surgeon because he made me feel listened to. We discussed my fears, worries, and concerns about having surgery as well as my hopes and desires for my changed nose. Based on his portfolio, I could see he did completely natural-looking work, and I wanted subtle and natural changes. I wanted my nose, but better. I trusted him completely. I wouldn't have gone through with it otherwise, no matter how much I may have wanted to change my nose.

I was excited waiting for the time of my surgery to finally arrive (I booked it three months ahead). The week before, I started to get unexpectedly nervous. Never was I nervous about the outcome because I trusted my surgeon. It was just the idea of going under anesthesia for two to three hours by choice! I wondered if I was being irresponsible. People in the world had surgery every day because they had to. But even if I had been able to cancel the surgery and get my money back, I wouldn't have. I was scared but did it anyway. A whole lifetime of waiting outweighed my worries about going under anesthesia.

Since I've had this done (it's only been two weeks, by the way), I've been thrilled. The amazing thing is that apparently it's only going to keep getting better for a while as the swelling (not noticeable, really) continues to go down over the next few weeks.

So it's like Christmas every day, looking in the mirror. No more catching my reflection here and there in some window or mirror and thinking "yuck," seeing that bump and pointy nose that I always wanted to hide behind my hand. Since my surgery, I've unexpectedly caught my reflection. My automatic reaction of thinking "yuck" would be at the ready in that split second before I realized that I liked what I saw. That's an incredibly liberating feeling. Now I can just be me.

Those last lines resonate with me. Sarah describes a feeling of liberation, a newfound freedom. She made the journey and can now just be herself. In Sarah, I see an example of someone who's successfully moved from what she considered an unacceptable group to an acceptable one.

LAUREL

When you finally correct a nose that's been troubling you for the better part of your life, the change can be dramatic. There's usually a period of adjustment in which you gradually come to see your new self as the real you—the you that was there all along, waiting to emerge. It can get a little confusing, as Laurel found out three months after her revision rhinoplasty.

I was at a wedding reception the other day, and a friend was roaming around, taking candid pictures on her digital camera.

At one point, she returned to show me the pictures she'd taken. A couple of the photos were of a group of our friends, chatting and laughing. I recognized all of them but one.

"Who's that?" I asked, puzzled.

She looked at me oddly, then realized I was serious.

"It's you," she said with a big grin.

I was shocked. I looked closer, and sure enough, the woman whose profile I couldn't identify was me.

After thirty-nine years, I finally look normal—and that's everything I'd hoped for.

MATTHEW

Matthew's story is remarkable for how he isolates and identifies the subtle changes that take place after rhinoplasty. You feel better about yourself, and that's reflected in your behavior. You become more open to others. People sense that and respond accordingly. They aren't reacting to your nose job; they're reacting to your reaction to it.

I'm a forty-four-year-old male psychiatrist. Please don't hold this against me, as I'm just a regular guy. I've always wished that my nose was different. My father is French Canadian, and he always made critical comments that I had the big French Canadian nose. I found those comments very hurtful.

When I was a little boy, I was on a teeter-totter with my twin brother. I remember flying off and banging my nose against it. Since then, my big nose had been deviated. I could breathe out of only one side.

Most people, however, felt I was good-looking enough in spite of my worries. A slightly displaced nose, a large nose, or even a receding hairline made no difference to how they felt about me. I felt generally the same way. I don't care about other people's appearances—and very few of us are Vogue or GQ model types.

What made me change my mind? I had a cancer scare. As a forty-year-old man, I had a PSA test (a blood test for prostate cancer). The results were alarming. I was diagnosed with prostate cancer in 2001.

I really started to reflect that life is truly short and that we all should do what we want to do. That was one aspect of it. The other was that I'm really struggling with the aging process. I really feel that, as I get older, I'm less attractive. My hair was falling out and losing its color. It's a transition in your life, and you really begin to wonder if anyone will find you attractive and, probably on a bigger scale, lovable.

I eventually decided to have the nose operation as I realize that life is precious for us all and the only real regrets in my life were for things I hadn't done or acted upon.

When I went back to work in two weeks, lots of people were impressed, though I still had some swelling. This was a good start. Over the next few weeks, I found myself looking into the mirror a lot and was fascinated in that I *could see the difference. I found that I was extremely happy and felt different about myself.*

As a psychiatrist, I had honestly thought that some, but not all, people have unrealistic expectations of how they'll feel about themselves after surgery. I'd also felt that some people have unrealistic expectations of how life will change for them or for how others will treat them. My experience was different than what I had anticipated. I found that I really did feel better about myself. I felt more attractive, confident, and interested in my appearance. I bought new clothes. I found myself able to laugh and enjoy things to an extent that I hadn't done in years. I felt much more playful and alive.

I emphasize that this procedure to alter my appearance made me feel much better about myself. I felt that it gave me a new look for my forties. It was clear to me that other people picked up on my happiness and actually did treat me differently. If people sense you feel good about yourself, this is an appealing quality to them. I was blown away that, even though I'm a psychiatrist, I had forgotten that anything is possible and that there's a difference between what you think and what you feel.

I do have some real sadness and regret that I chose not to have the surgery in my younger years. I wish I had made the decision to have the surgery in my thirties.

This experience with the nose job has reinforced for me that I'm worthy of treating myself well, that the only real regrets in my life are for things that I wish I had done, and that the way you feel about yourself influences the way you treat others and the way others treat you in return.

CHRISTINA

Christina's journey took her into the perilous territory of family disapproval. She comes from a large and proud family of Italian descent. Strong facial features, including prominent noses, are seen within the family as an integral part of their identity. Wanting to change that seemed like an insult to them, as though Christina were rejecting her kin.

I took the plunge and had a primary rhinoplasty in May of 2003. It still amazes me to this day that I actually went through with this surgery. It was one of the most difficult decisions I've ever had to make.

I've always hated my nose, probably since puberty, but never really considered plastic surgery very seriously. Then one day, a friend of mine brought her wedding pictures into work. As I was flipping through them, I came across a couple of pictures that the photographer had managed to take of my profile. As I stared at the pictures in front of me, all I could see was how terrible my nose looked and how it didn't seem to fit in with the rest of my facial features. I realized for the first time that I didn't have to live with my nose this way. I could easily improve the appearance of my nose with plastic surgery.

Now that I was seriously considering having surgery, I realized that I had a lot of things to take into account. I needed to find the right doctor with the right credentials. I met with three surgeons before ultimately deciding on Dr. Adamson. I wanted someone who specialized in the face and had extensive experience. I had complete trust in

Dr. Adamson from the beginning. He was very open and honest with me about what he felt he could accomplish with surgery. He explained to me that his goal wasn't to make me look like a completely different person but more like a refreshed version of myself.

I also realized in meeting with Dr. Adamson that I needed to have realistic expectations about the outcome of my surgery. No doctor is perfect, so I couldn't expect perfection. That was a scary reality for me in the beginning, but I trusted my decision and was confident in Dr. Adamson's abilities.

Having said all that, it still wasn't an easy decision for me to make. From the time that I booked the surgery until the day of surgery I felt like I was on an emotional roller coaster. Even on the day of surgery, I wasn't 100 percent sure that this was the right decision for me, but I knew that if I didn't go through with it, I'd regret it for the rest of my life.

I received a lot of opposition from my family and friends. They thought it was ridiculous that I wanted to change something that had been part of me for over twenty-four years. They felt that I should forget about the surgery and concentrate on what they believed were the more important things in my life. They had the notion that I believed I'd be a better person somehow if I had the surgery.

I explained to them that this wasn't the case. I didn't want the surgery because I thought more people would like me, or I'd be prettier, or because I thought I'd get more attention. I wanted this surgery for me, for my own satisfaction, and for my own sanity. I wanted to never have to think about my nose again, and if I did, I wanted my thoughts to be good ones.

My family eventually realized that my intentions were sincere and that, though they didn't understand my decision, it was something that was extremely important to me in my life.

In the months before surgery, I used the Internet to gather more information. I came across a few facial plastic surgery forums, where I received a lot of information and support. On one of these sites, I met a girl who was also considering rhinoplasty. We made a connection and hit it off instantly. Our friendship turned out to be a strong support for me throughout the entire process. I had someone to turn to who completely understood what I was going through and could relate to any fears or excitements that I had. It's truly amazing how our friendship has developed from one common thread. Both of us had surgery with Dr. Adamson on the exact same day. It's funny sometimes how people are brought together under the most unusual circumstances.

My recovery has been wonderful. The changes I see in the pictures that I've taken throughout my recovery are amazing and fascinating. The surgery hasn't changed who I am or what I believe in; it has only changed the way I look. The part I like most about my results is that they're very natural. I still look like me, just a better version of myself—and this is what the ultimate goal of plastic surgery is. I'm definitely more comfortable now in a lot of situations. I seldom think about my nose anymore, and when I do, they're pleasant thoughts. I don't care now if people take pictures of my profile because it's absolutely beautiful. On my wedding day, I won't be thinking about the angle the photographer is taking the picture from; I'll be thinking only of how lucky I am to be marrying the man of my dreams.

Some still believe that it's a shame that it took cosmetic surgery to make me feel this way about myself, but I'm not in the least ashamed or embarrassed that I did this. I'm proud that I had the strength and the courage to undergo such a procedure to improve myself.

This has been a very positive experience for me. I can't find the words to express how happy I am that I decided to have this surgery or to explain how thrilled I am with my results.

Happily, Christina's family is coming to terms with her rhinoplasty. They now realize that it wasn't about rejection of them but about Christina's acceptance of herself.

SUSAN

Some patients are list-makers, and that's generally a good thing. When Susan saw me about her nose, she'd clearly done her homework. She came prepared with many questions. All doctors find that patients can only absorb so much information during a consultation. This, of course, is especially true when you're getting bad news about your health. You remember the diagnosis with great clarity ("Oh my God, I've got cancer"), but the information that follows is a fog. This, to a lesser extent, is also true of people who come in for cosmetic surgery. You just can't absorb it all. That's why we always follow up with further meetings and plenty of printed information.

But it's also a good idea to bring someone with you to your consultation to make notes. But if you're like Susan, you may just make those notes on your own.

I guess you could call me nose-obsessed. I examine just about every nose I meet. With the best noses, I try to find some telltale sign of a nose job, anything to encourage my obsession. I've been known to approach total strangers with "You have a great nose," hoping this would spur on some rhino rhetoric. I'm actually pretty good at spotting a "done" nose. I've also come across some sad stories of rhinoplasty gone wrong. I've learned that cosmetic nasal surgery is the most difficult of all cosmetic surgeries.

I knew I needed the best surgeon I could find. There was much at stake—the risk of an unsuccessful outcome. I decided I'd decrease that risk by having only the best nose doctor operate on me. But how to find that surgeon? I began by researching on the Internet and became a regular on rhino-plasty discussion boards. Certain names cropped up, includ-ing Dr. Adamson's. I checked out his website and then phoned his office. I had a few questions. How many rhinoplasties did he perform a year? (about one hundred, I was told) Did he perform revisions? (yes) Did he revise other surgeons' work? (yes) I figured that a good revisionist would perform an excel-lent primary. What was his personal rate of revision? (about 5 percent) My questions were treated with such respect by the staff that I felt comfortable asking anything.

My first consultation with Dr. Adamson would be in a month and a half. I couldn't wait to meet him. I was so excited on the day of my consultation that I felt like I was going on a first date. What if he didn't like me? Worse yet, what if he didn't like my nose?

Dr. Adamson met me with a big smile and a firm handshake. I had a list of questions a mile long. By the end of the consultation, he'd answered just about every question I had without my even having to ask. He had this way of referring to my nose as "our nose." He described how he would reshape my nose to highlight my strong features. I was in total agreement with everything he suggested: bring down the slight bump, refine and raise the droopy tip, and improve my breathing by straightening my deviated septum. We weren't aiming for perfection, only a nice improvement.

On the day of the surgery, I was extremely excited and nervous and had to keep reminding myself to stay in the moment and try to remember every detail. I was finally going through with it! I couldn't believe it!

I was surprisingly talkative and remember telling the anesthesiologist, "I'm feeling better and better all the time." And then I was out.

When I woke up, I felt groggy, sleepy, and nauseated. Through my haze, I managed to croak, "How did it go?" I was told that everything had gone perfectly, and then I fell happily back to sleep. I remember thinking how incredible it was that, after all this time and all this planning, it was finally over. But what was under my cast? I was so excited to see the final results.

The next week was difficult. The nausea continued for a couple of days, and I was pretty miserable and very emotional. There was surprisingly little pain, but the bruising and swelling made up for that. Luckily, I was well-prepared for what to expect after surgery. Still, seeing myself in the cast and bandages with two black eyes, my face swollen like a chipmunk, was hard.

I was so worried about the possibility of bumping my new nose that I slept with a huge pillow separating my husband and me. No one was allowed within three feet of my nose. My sister-in-law was kind enough to take care of my three-year-old daughter for a week. My ten-year-old son was permitted to live at home with extreme caution.

At the end of the week, my daughter returned home. She'd been warned of my condition. When she first set eyes on me, cast and all, she was sweet enough to say that I must look like a fairy princess under my bandages.

Finally, seven days post-op, came the unveiling. I was so anxious to see my new nose. When the cast came off, I was still swollen but could see the improvement. I loved the shape of my new nose.

At six weeks post-op, my nose continued to refine. As time went on, it began to feel more and more like a part of me.

At eight weeks after the surgery, my columellar scar was nearly invisible. No one would have been able to tell that I had ever had an operation on my nose.

I'm now ten weeks into my healing and haven't regretted my decision to have rhinoplasty for an instant. I now have the nose I should have been born with.

Susan's journey had its moments of high emotion and low misery but ended happily—with the nose she felt she should have had all along. Of all the procedures that we cosmetic facial surgeons do, rhinoplasty can be the most transformative.

KIMBERLY

Kimberly the nurse always referred to the protrusion on the front of her face not as a nose but as a "defect." As an adolescent, she found herself in purgatory, not just ignored by the boys but actually taunted by them. "You're so ugly," they had said right to her stricken face. That kind of unthinking cruelty can leave lasting emotional scars. That was the case with Kim. I have much admiration for her strength in dealing with it.

For most of my adult life, I've been painfully self-conscious of a nasal defect that resulted from a poorly done previous surgery.

People would stare at my nose, ask me questions about it, and, since it was obvious that I had had surgery on it, offer suggestions as to how it should be fixed.

I dreaded situations in which people could observe my nose. Cocktail parties were a nightmare. When I rode the subway, I was always aware of the people sitting on either side, possibly studying my "unusual" profile. I'd try to find a seat at the end of a subway car or at the back of a bus or classroom—anywhere that I couldn't be seen from the side. When I walked down the street, I looked at the ground rather than encounter the stares of strangers.

Although I'm a friendly person and work well in my health care profession with the patients in my care, I was reluctant to make professional presentations or to put forward ideas before groups of colleagues because I felt that people were staring at my defect. My natural shyness became terribly exaggerated.

I was constantly aware of my nose. The only place I felt comfortable was in the privacy of my own home. Even there, whenever I looked into a mirror to style my hair or apply makeup, I was reminded of my defect.

In my fifties, I became unhappy with forehead furrows and jowls developing in my face. I went online to research plastic surgery of the face and found photos of people before and after having had face-lifts. When I found Dr. Adamson's website and read his mission statement, I felt confident he was the right surgeon to do the surgery on me. In fact, I remembered that he'd been recommended to me years earlier by another well-known plastic surgeon in Toronto. I immediately made an appointment.

During my consultation, I found that he and his staff made me feel totally comfortable—no small accomplishment since we were discussing the very defect upon which I least wanted attention.

I had no reservations about either the face-lift or the nasal revision surgery.

As for the nasal revision, it's radically improved my life. I no longer limit my activities according to how I may be seen by others. I go wherever I want, sit wherever I please, and speak up in a crowd if I want to. I feel normal for the first time in my life.

No one suspects I've had surgery, but I've been asked by various people if I've been on an extended vacation, changed my hairstyle, or lost weight. People remark on the improvement but can't put their finger on exactly what has happened. I'm still me, only better and fresher. I really feel that for the rest of my life, the sky's the limit.

JILLIAN

Jillian had broken her nose several times and had trouble breathing. She was also unhappy with how it looked and made her feel about herself. Surgery helped her with both these issues.

Since my teens, I had been unhappy with my nose. I felt self-conscious when people looked at me from the side, as I thought my nose looked ugly. Years of competitive downhill skiing and other sports had caused injuries to my nose (and breakage of other bones on various occasions). My mother had urged me to wait until my twenties to have surgery, as she felt that my face was still developing and changing.

Finally, I felt as though I had waited long enough to see that the shape of my nose wasn't going to change on its own. Additionally, I rarely breathed through my nose since it never seemed to supply me with enough oxygen. This bothered me.

Since my surgery, I feel as though my life has changed in both noticeable and subtle ways. Most noticeable to me are that I can breathe through my nose with ease and that my nose looks attractive to me for the first time in my adult life. On a more subtle level, I no longer cringe when I see profile pictures of myself. I feel more positive, self-confident, and happy in my life. I feel more beautiful.

ANNE

Anne's is another family story. Anne is very close to her dad. She inherited his quick wit, his curiosity about life, his agile mind—and his nose.

My nose seemed to keep growing after the rest of me stopped. Bigger and bigger—or at least, that's how I felt as a fifteen-year-old. That feeling dulled a bit as I got older, but it didn't go away.

Fear of a bad or unnatural-looking result was the only thing that kept me from getting it fixed, and for years, I lived with it. For others in the same boat, you know how it feels to turn your head away when waiting at a red light in traffic so that the complete stranger in the next car can't see your nose in profile! It's this self-consciousness that I'm happy to get rid of, more than the big nose itself.

At thirty, I decided to take the plunge. After a lot of research, I went through with the surgery. It was a frightening prospect; even though after talking to many former patients and feeling sure my surgeon would do a great job, there was still that scary sensation of not knowing what the outcome would be.

The day of surgery, I felt like I was jumping off a cliff, just totally letting go with fingers tightly crossed, hoping for the best.

I needn't have worried, as the following week, my nose and chin implant (to balance out the profile) were revealed. Despite the swelling and slight bruising, I could tell I was going to be thrilled. What a relief that was.

Now, ten months later, it feels like I've always had this nose. I think it's almost funny how anxious and apprehensive I was about the surgery. A life lived in fear is a life half-lived.

That feeling of finally having the "right" nose usually comes a few months after rhinoplasty. I have patients who report that they now have to look at old photographs to remember what they looked like before surgery. It's as though they've forgotten what they used to look like. I think what happens is that when we improve the things they don't like (such as a bump or bulbous tip), they feel they're finally the way they always should have been.

Some psychologists would say, "Well, that's too bizarre. That shouldn't be. What you are is what you are." Others would say you should be happy with your appearance because it's what God gave you. But the reality is that people think of themselves with their nicer noses as looking the way they were meant to look. This is the real them. And they get into that new feeling very quickly.

CHAPTER SIXTEEN

We soon learn that there is nothing mysterious or supernatural in the case, but that all proceeds from the usual propensity of mankind toward the marvelous.

— *David Hume,* philosopher

HEALING TOUCH

When we talk about healing, what do we really mean? The ancient root of the word means "to make whole." In modern Western medicine, that usually consists of finding and employing a medical treatment for a diagnosed biological ailment. That's fine as far as it goes, but could there be more? Many doctors are turning to other measures, not to replace medical treatments but to complement them. They're exploring the other side of medicine: the alternative side, with its emphasis on treating the patient as a whole person—body, mind, and spirit. What was once dismissed as mysticism is now being embraced as an exciting and often effective way to promote healing, reduce discomfort, and manage stress.

Increasing numbers of doctors are introducing mind- and energy-oriented therapies, such as meditation, reflexology, and massage, into the operating theater and recovery room. On the surface, such therapies may seem New Age and trendy, and perhaps a little suspicious. But they've been around for ages. Many of these therapies were established in ancient Eastern cultures. Some doctors and other practitioners call this combination of alternative and Western approaches "integrative medicine."

HEALING TOUCH

One of the most interesting modalities, and the one that caught my attention, is called Healing Touch. It uses energy-based healing to reduce anxiety and to help patients look better sooner after surgery and have less discomfort. Practitioners apply Healing Touch to the energy field that surrounds the body and even to the energy centers within the body. It's totally noninvasive. The practitioner uses his or her hands to clear, energize, and balance the human and environmental energy fields around the patient. The aim is to effect physical, emotional, mental, and spiritual health and healing.

It seems to work for some patients. Over the last two decades, the use of energy-based healing in modern medicine has gained wide acceptance because of anecdotal reports of its effectiveness. Research into the healing influence of the human energy field has prompted many universities to establish professional training for nurses in holistic healing. Leading North American hospitals are incorporating energy-based therapies into their postoperative treatments.

It is reasonable to expect the doctor to recognize that science may not have all the answers to problems of health and healing.

—*Norman Cousins*, journalist and professor

Some cosmetic facial surgeons, including me, are doing the same thing. In my experience, energy-based healing has its place for selected patients throughout the process of cosmetic surgery. It seems to help relieve patient stress and anxiety before the operation, and it may speed the healing process in the days and weeks after surgery for some people.

Consider this: You've decided, after much deliberation, to have a face-lift. You're understandably anxious about it, perhaps more than anxious. You may be fearful. As the day of your surgery approaches, all the research you've done and all the preparations you've gone through, including preoperative consultations with your surgeon, don't seem to matter. You're worried sick and feel as though you can't do anything about it except grit your teeth and plunge ahead or turn tail and run for the door.

Now, in the hour or so before the operation, you spend time with a Healing Touch practitioner and find yourself less anxious, even relaxed, as you enter surgery. Afterward, the bruising, though present, isn't as great as expected. Furthermore, the healing process moves along a little more quickly than expected.

CLEARWELL RAPID RECOVERY SYSTEM
That's what happened to Bonita when she had her face-lift. She was very nervous about the procedure—unusually so—but had made the fully informed decision to press on.

Bonita's surgery was in my hands, but I shared another aspect of her care with someone else. Susan Morales is not only a qualified nurse but also a nursing instructor and a pioneer in complementary therapy education and research. She's a specialist in the growing field of holistic nursing and the founder of the Clearwell Rapid Recovery System.

How does it work? It's essentially a mind-body treatment regimen specifically tailored for people undergoing plastic surgery. Susan begins the process by working with patients in their homes to help them relax and to prepare emotionally for surgery using visualization techniques, an effective and time-honored way to relieve stress.

Now she adds an energy treatment that will be repeated during and after surgery. It's called biofield therapy, and it involves working with the invisible energy field believed to exist around the human body. Using her hands, Susan scans the body from head to toe, picking up differences in the energy level and going through a process called "clearing." With a gentle waving motion, her hands clear and smooth disturbances in the energy field. This process can also go on during surgery and in the recovery room.

The process is based on the practitioner and client coming together energetically to facilitate the client's health and healing. The goal is to restore harmony and balance in the energy system, placing the client in a position to self-heal. It complements conventional health care and is used in collaboration with other approaches to health and healing. Some of it is based on tried-and-true relaxation techniques, including visualization. Close your eyes, plant your feet squarely on the floor, breathe deeply, and create a mental picture of your favorite tranquil place—your garden, or a quiet beach on a summer day. Already, you're feeling calmer and more relaxed.

Its principal aim is to reduce emotional tension and stress in the patient. But there's a second goal: to reduce stress on the body (that is, the actual surgical stress on tissue). Any kind of surgery is a shock to the system. In facial plastic surgery, you expect to see postoperative puffiness, bruising, and swelling. The body's natural defences and built-in healing mechanisms go to work, and the healing process begins.

With Healing Touch, the kind of therapy employed by Susan Morales and her team of practitioners, that process (in some cases) doesn't seem to take as long. In short, there's some evidence that Healing Touch enables a cosmetic surgery patient to experience less bruising and swelling and return to normal more quickly. We haven't yet been able to prove this scientifically, but anecdotally, we've had many patients who have benefitted from their Healing Touch experience.

Susan Morales, R.N., M.S.N., C.H.T.I.

Healing Touch is a biofield therapy. That means we work with the energy field around the human body, the biofield. It's based on the principle that the practitioner can assess that energy field. It's usually done with the hands, but it may not be just the hands. It can be a high sense perception— actually seeing. It could be auditory.

The human energy field has four basic layers, but there's one that's the exact double of the physical body, and it extends about two to four inches (five to ten centimeters) away. It's called the etheric field or vital field.

*As we scan the body from head to toe, we pick up dif-
ferences. Then, as we dialogue with the client, we see if
there's a problem in that area, or why our attention may be
drawn to it. Based on the assessment, we then choose a specific technique and use it as an intervention. Afterward, we
re-evaluate to see what has shifted energetically in the field.
We also get feedback from the client.*

*Are we accurate all the time? Of course not. I've been
doing this for thirty years and tend to trust my intuitive
senses in my assessment. I'd say, from a spiritual sense—
and this is just me, personally—that there is a soul, and a
physical body within it. It isn't just a protein body with
molecules, hemoglobin, fluids, and tissue. We know that
there's an emotional domain, an intellectual domain, and a
spiritual domain.*

*Can I measure the energy field? Can I see it on an
MRI? No, but there are many phenomena that medical science cannot yet explain.*

*My dad is a hard-core science guy. His training was in
chemistry, but he became an M.D. He's pretty left-brained,
analytical, and skeptical. He had serious open-heart cardiac
surgery at the age of eighty-five. I did Healing Touch on
him for twelve hours a day, and he survived. He walked out
of the hospital. His doctors couldn't believe it.*

*My mother recently had shingles along the trigeminal
nerve. The shingles went, but now she suffers from something called post-herpetic neuralgia. It's very painful. I had
Healing Touch people treating her. I also taught my father*

how to do the move we call clearing the field or sweeping. He now believes that it really helped my mother. He's now very much a believer.

He's come a long way, as have a lot of medical people. The whole thing about complementary therapy has just opened up. The National Institutes of Health in the United States provide a lot of money for research funding through their National Center for Complementary and Alternative Medicine.

When I go into surgery with a client, I know that the minute the surgery begins, I'm helping with the energy flow. There has been cutting, a break in the integrity of the subtle levels of the energy field, so I help with the reintegration. Swelling and bruising is a natural phenomenon. What I'm trying to do is to optimize that natural physiological response in the quickest amount of time to facilitate their healing. What we're finding is that people I've worked with are not that swollen and not that bruised. I think that has to do with the preparation. Perhaps the shock to the body isn't so great, or the body is better able to deal with it because there has been prep. How much faster do people recover? I won't put a number to it, like 50 percent faster, because each person is different. But I will say that I believe Healing Touch does make a difference for people having cosmetic surgery.

The skeptic in all of us asks, "Where's the proof?" The evidence of the effectiveness of Healing Touch in cosmetic surgery is so far anecdotal. We have seen patients who seem to do better with the backup or complementary aid of Healing Touch.

I believe that alternative treatments have their place in modern Western medicine and particularly in cosmetic surgery. I find Clearwell Rapid Recovery to be an exciting and progressive addition to our list of restorative services. Time and further study will, we hope, help us ultimately determine the real effects of this kind of treatment.

CHAPTER SEVENTEEN

Life is a daring adventure or it is nothing at all.

— *Helen Keller,* author, activist, and lecturer

THE TRANSFORMATION

The day after your plastic surgery, you may think that you've made a huge, calamitous mistake, and that the face-lift or rhinoplasty was reckless and dumb.

PATIENTS' REACTIONS AFTER SURGERY

Valerie had her morning-after moment when she looked in the mirror, turned to her husband, and whispered, "My face turned into hamburger."

"No," he replied. "It's more like E.T."

Valerie had been summoning the courage to have a face-lift for years, and it had come down to this. She was being compared to a bug-eyed extraterrestrial. "Thanks a lot," she replied.

Arpi had the same "What have I gone and done?" experience. She was propped up in bed, a gauze bandage under her nose. "I was in all my bruised glory, black and blue, and I could barely open my eyes because they were so swollen," Arpi recalls.

Her husband came in with a camera. "Nobody's going to believe this," he said, taking a picture. "It looks like somebody beat the crap out of you."

"Very eloquently put, thank you very much," Arpi mumbled. "That makes me feel great."

Valerie and Arpi found solace in a cold washcloth on the eyes and a little irony on the tongue. Forgive them, in their morning-after miseries, for thinking it was all a big mistake, and that this was the worst thing they've ever done.

Check in a few weeks later, and the whole mood is considerably brighter.

Valerie: "If I had to make the decision again—face-lift, yes or no—you can bet the answer would be a resounding *yes.*"

Arpi: "My husband says, 'Oh, honey, you look fabulous,' and I say, 'That's all I wanted to hear.'"

THE REALITY OF TRANSFORMATION

People who have plastic surgery undergo a transformation—both physically and mentally. Negative feelings turn into positive ones. The journey begins with feelings of self-consciousness, embarrassment, or even shame. These feelings are followed by curiosity about making a change. Then comes the fear of going ahead and the inevitable guilt. A more positive range of feelings takes over, including excitement, courage, and hope, tempered by the morning-after "What have I done?" dip.

Plastic surgery is transformative, but it doesn't change people into something they're not. In reality, my patients feel that they're having the surgery to change themselves into what they really are.

My patients often tell me that they feel like they aren't part of the group of what they would consider normal-looking people.

They're not looking to cheat death or be better than everyone else. It's not about vanity. They don't want to look like celebrities or be in *Vogue* or *GQ*. They just want to become part of the crowd.

I believe that this is an important philosophical or psychological aspect of what plastic surgeons do. You need to understand the inner discomfort, anxiety, and (in some cases) emotional pain that drives people to undergo plastic surgery. There must be a strong psychological impetus to voluntarily allow someone to put a scalpel to your face.

I also believe that plastic surgery can have its own halo effect, generating unanticipated positive consequences. Guilt is one of the most common feelings that patients go through on the long journey. They ask themselves why they'd spend time and money on themselves when there's so much else in the world that needs fixing. In my experience, people who feel guilty before surgery usually don't feel guilty after surgery. In fact, because they feel better about themselves, they often contribute more to society. I strongly believe that if we all make the best we can of our own lives, we're making our whole society better.

People often report feeling physically better and more energetic after plastic surgery—not the day or even the week after, but a few months down the line. A recent study showed a measured increase in health-related quality of life among cosmetic facial surgery patients. While there were differences according to sex, age, and procedure, the largest increase in quality of life was in the category of general self-consciousness of appearance.

CHAPTER EIGHTEEN

THE OTHER FACES OF PLASTIC SURGERY

BABIDJANA

A little girl rides her bicycle down an urban street. Her name is Babidjana. There is little traffic and few pedestrians. It's quiet, unusually so. Without warning, the tranquility is shattered by gunfire. The child looks up—and in that instant, her life is changed forever.

A bullet ricochets off a lamppost and hits her in the face.

This is Grozny, the capital of Chechnya, in 1999. The fighting between Chechen rebels and the Russian military is about to flare up again. Before it's over, Grozny will be reduced to rubble.

Babidjana lies in the street beside her bike. The gunmen disappear. An ambulance takes her to the hospital. She's one of half a million child victims of the Chechen fighting. There is no accurate casualty count. The plight of those who escape the bombs and bullets is measured in appalling rates of malnutrition, tuberculosis, intestinal infections, hepatitis A, whooping cough, mumps, and measles. The psychological trauma is immeasurable. This is the collateral damage of war.

Babidjana might be willing to endure all this misery in exchange for the horror that has befallen her—and for what lies ahead. The bullet tore away half of her face. The doctors in Grozny can do little but stabilize her and deliver her into the hands of what many of them consider the enemy.

Babidjana is airlifted deep into Russia, to Yekaterinburg in the Ural Mountains, the last stop on the way to Siberia. This is an industrial city, one of the off-limits places of the old Soviet Union. No one, and certainly no foreigner, could get in without special permission. It was here in 1918 that Bolshevik revolutionaries assassinated the Russian czar and his family in the ominously named "house of special purpose."

Here Babidjana finds herself in one of the most heartbreaking places on the planet, a crowded orphanage populated with maimed, deformed, and unwanted children. They're the victims of traumatic and congenital conditions. Some have been left here by parents too poor to take care of them. And some, like Babidjana, are the casualties of war.

The orphanage is part of the Bonum Centre, a surgical institute for pediatric deformities. Here, a staff of skilled plastic surgeons, anesthesiologists, and nurses, working in years past with limited and outdated equipment, do their best to repair the broken faces of the children. It was here that Babidjana had her face rebuilt. Her injuries were horrendous. The bullet had shattered her cheek and jaw. The operation took the better part of a day.

IVAN C.

Down the hall from Babidjana, a Russian boy, Ivan C., is about to begin an ordeal that will take him through four reconstructive surgeries over five years. He was born with a cleft lip, a clubfoot, and deformed limbs. He was also born deaf, the victim of chronic serous otitis media, a buildup of fluid in the middle ear. That meant he faced the prospect of never learning to speak.

When Ivan's mother learned of all the surgery he would need, she abandoned him to the orphanage—and then left the rest of her family and moved out of the country. She believed the child was mentally retarded, but no one ever made this diagnosis.

This is the other face of plastic surgery. Every year, a team of North American doctors goes to Yekaterinburg to work with our Russian counterparts on the faces of children who are considered unadoptable because of their deformities.

THE BONUM CENTRE

This isn't so-called parachute medicine, where we go in and take over. It's a collaborative effort with the Bonum Centre surgeons. They're skilled professionals but operate under dire conditions. There isn't enough equipment, and medications are always in short supply. On one facial reconstruction case, the respirator overheated and failed. The Russian doctor assisting me had to blow through a tube to ventilate the young patient.

Whatever you can do, or dream you can, begin it. Boldness has genius, power and magic in it.

– attributed to Wolfgang von Goethe, philosopher

Over the years, we've performed more than 600 operations at
the Bonum Centre. We see cleft lips and palates, deformed ears,
facial paralysis, tumors, and worse. A common problem is reti-
nopathy of the premature, a condition that can lead to blind-
ness in infants. It's treatable if found in time and, for that
reason, is rare in North America and Western Europe. But it's
widespread in this poor part of Russia. On one mission to
Yekaterinburg, we had an eye specialist who showed the Russian doctors how to identify and treat this disease. As a result,
the number of blind children at the orphanage has begun to
decrease.

There's give-and-take here. We share our expertise with
our Russian colleagues. In return, we get to extend our skills
as plastic and reconstructive surgeons beyond the cosmetic.
We see things we've never seen before—and wish we never had
to. One seven-year-old boy had been in the orphanage most of
his life, given up as a baby after a rat came into his crib and
chewed off his nose. We reconstructed the nose, using techniques that hadn't been seen in Russia before. It will have to be
repeated when the boy reaches adolescence. The Yekaterinburg surgeons now have the knowledge to do it. They learn the
latest reconstructive surgery techniques from us. From them,
we learn how the Bonum Centre's staff's dedication and commitment provide hope and a better future for the children in
their care. This whole area of medicine is further along in
Europe and North America than in the far reaches of Russia,
where simply keeping young patients alive is the day-to-day
challenge.

HAPPY ENDINGS

There's a survival-of-the-fittest reality to life here that many in the West would probably find disturbing. The sad fact is that parents, especially the heads of families living in poverty, can't cope with deformed children. It's not surprising that most of the newly arrived children have problems that go well beyond the physical. Many are withdrawn and slow to develop. Some don't, or can't, speak. They all hope to find families. Progress here is measured in small increments.

Case number 4982 is an example of what I'm talking about. Boris S. was born in 1998 with both a cleft lip and palate, and was abandoned by his parents. The mid-part of Boris's upper lip wasn't there, and there was a hole in the roof of his mouth. He arrived at the orphanage in a precarious state, suffering from birth defects and rickets, a disease that causes softening of the bones. In this case, it had already produced some deformity in his arms and legs. In 1999, we surgically corrected Boris' cleft lip and palate. He's still living at the orphanage.

So is Ivan K., case 3688. Ivan, born in 1991, has had four operations to repair a cleft lip and palate. His social worker reports that he's now very sociable and has many friends. The boy has come out of his shell. At the orphanage, this is a triumph. But, as of this writing, Ivan still doesn't have a family.

Others are luckier. Boris C. had essentially the same problem, corrected by operations in 1998 and 1999. In 2004, he was adopted and now lives in the United States. Dimitry, after two operations, was adopted by a family in Switzerland. He now lives in Bern and plays hockey and guitar. "He has no problems with learning language," writes Dimitry's case worker. "He's very active in communicating with people and has many friends. He's doing well in school."

There are some happy endings. Babidjana was returned to her family in Chechnya. Ivan C., whose mother believed he was mentally challenged, was reunited with his father.

FACE TO FACE

These are some of the people we've encountered on our trips to Russia. The program, called FACE TO FACE, has been going since 1992. It was founded by the American Academy of Facial Plastic and Reconstructive Surgery (AAFPRS), which also supports humanitarian medical missions to many other parts of the world. In 1996, one of my grateful and very generous patients helped us to create the Canadian Foundation for Facial Plastic and Reconstructive Surgery to support our missions. Together with our American counterparts, we (along with surgeons and nurses from many parts of the world) have performed surgeries on children in Russia, China, Cuba, Bosnia, Southest Asia, and Central America.

The work in Yekaterinburg has shown gratifying results. More than eighty children have had restorative surgery and have been either adopted or returned to their families. Year by year, it continues and is in constant need of support. Everything, it seems, is always in short supply.

Happily, in recent years there has been increased funding for the Bonum Centre, allowing expansion to more modern facilities and more children to be served. Our mission now also travels to Saratov, Russia, and plans are underway to send missions to other countries as well.

I believe that it's important to share professional knowledge, to pass on some of the things I've learned to other doctors. But the most satisfying part of this work is helping the children. My mother was right: You get more from what you give than from what you take.

CHAPTER NINETEEN

All truths are easy to understand once they are discovered. The trick is to discover them.

– *Galileo Galilei,* astronomer

A FINAL WORD

What now?

You've had a glimpse at what it's really like to have cosmetic facial surgery. You've seen from my patients' stories that it's not about transforming yourself into someone different but about revealing who you really are. It's about having your outer appearance reflect your inner self and the goal of achieving a natural, "unoperated" look.

I hope that the stories my patients were kind enough to share with you will help you to make your decision.

You may be ready to take the journey. If so, remember that it's a step-by-step process. Be sure to give it all the care and attention that it deserves. Be frank with yourself about what you believe needs to be changed, whether it's an aging face, a misshapen nose, or some other problem. Talk to people who have had work done. Try to put your worries and concerns into perspective. Take care in choosing your doctor.

Above all, remember that this is your decision and your journey. You're responsible for your own future and making your life the best it can be for you.

GLOSSARY

autograft: Tissue removed from one place in the body and inserted into another area of the body for reconstructive purposes. For instance, cartilage may be taken from the ear or nasal septum to reconstruct the nose.

banding: Vertical bands of excess skin and/or sagging muscle in the neck, usually due to aging.

blepharoplasty: Cosmetic surgery of the upper and lower eyes. Tiny amounts of skin are removed to correct "hooding" in the upper eyelids. Fat is removed from or repositioned beneath the lower lids to reduce or eliminate the saggy, pouchy look.

Botox: Trade name for botulinum toxin. When injected, it temporarily weakens the muscles in the face that, over time, have caused deep furrows between the eyes, across the forehead, in the crow's feet, or in other areas. Botox injections are usually repeated every few months.

botulinum toxin: Generic name for Botox.

brow lift: Surgery to restore a more youthful look to the area above the eyes. Several surgical approaches are available, including minimally invasive endoscopic surgery, to elevate eyebrows and reduce forehead wrinkles.

canula: Slender tube used in liposuction. It is inserted beneath the skin and moved around to loosen and remove fat deposits by suction.

cheiloplasty: Lip augmentation or reduction surgery.

chemical peel: Resurfacing the skin with an acid solution that peels the top layer and allows smoother, regenerated skin to emerge. Many different solutions and strengths are available.

cheek augmentation: *See* **malarplasty.**

chin augmentation: *See* **genioplasty.**

closed rhinoplasty: Nasal surgery performed through incisions inside the nose. It is often used for less complicated procedures. Also called *endonasal rhinoplasty.*

collagen: The fibrous protein constituent of skin, cartilage, bone, and other connective tissue. More than a third of the body's protein, and more than 75 percent of skin, is collagen. It is also used in fillers.

cording: *See* **banding.**

coronal forehead lift: A brow lift that involves an ear-to-ear incision over the top of the scalp, cutting some muscles in the forehead and pulling up tissue under the skin to eliminate lines.

deep plane face-lift: A face-lift in which the level of dissection is taken below the SMAS (superficial musculoaponeurotic system) and platysma muscle, allowing not only a skin lift but also a lift of the facial muscles and fascia. Several modifications are available, depending on specific patient needs.

dermabrasion: Facial sanding technique for deep scars and wrinkles, raised scar tissue, and severe cystic acne. Top layers of skin are "sanded" off with a high-speed rotating brush or a diamond-coated wheel. Laser treatments have replaced many of the traditional uses of dermabrasion.

ear pinning: *See* **otoplasty.**

electrocautery: Using an electric current through a fine needle or forceps to treat skin lesions or to stop bleeding.

electrolysis: Treatment of hair roots by electric action through a fine needle.

ePTFE: Expanded polytetrafluoroethylene. It is the chemical name for Goretex, a durable, inert substance used in nasal and other implants.

endoscope: A small, cylindrical surgical telescope inserted through an incision or orifice to diagnose and operate. It enables the performance of minimally invasive surgery.

endoscopic forehead lift: Elevation of the eyebrows through small incisions behind the hairline.

endoscopic midface lift: Elevation of the cheeks through a small incision behind the temple hairline.

eyelid lift: *See* **blepharoplasty.**

external rhinoplasty: *See* **open rhinoplasty.**

face-lift: *See* **rhytidectomy.**

facial peel: *See* **chemical peel.**

facial plastic surgery: Specialized plastic surgery of the face, both cosmetic and reconstructive. It is also the name of the surgical specialty that carries out such surgery.

fascia: Firm, non-elastic tissue beneath the skin in the cheeks that is modified in a face-lift. It is also known as *SMAS fascia*.

fillers: Substances injected into the face to smooth out creases or wrinkles. They are used primarily in the lower face, especially in the creases that run from the side of the nose to the mouth and in the lips and fine lines around the mouth. They are also very effective in adding lost tissue volume back into the face, especially to correct sagging cheeks and the furrow in front of the jowls. Dozens of fillers are available. Most, such as Juvéderm and Restylane, are temporary, lasting six to nine months in the lips and nine months or longer in larger facial creases. Permanent fillers consist of microscopic plasticized material suspended in collagen. When injected, the collagen is absorbed into the body, leaving the permanent material in place.

flap: Skin tissue that is moved from one place to another close by to reconstruct a defect, keeping part of the skin attached (the flap pedicle) to maintain its blood supply.

forehead lift: *See* **brow lift.**

generic name: The nonproprietary name for a drug.

genioplasty: Chin augmentation.

Goretex: Trade name of ePTFE (expanded polytetrafluoroethylene), a dorsal nasal implant.

graft: Tissue (such as cartilage or skin) that is separated from its blood supply, moved to another place in the body for reconstruction, and lives through the growth of its new blood supply.

head and neck surgery: *See* **otolaryngology.**

hooding: Sagging of the skin of the upper eyes, causing an aging and tired look. It can be due to sagging brows and/or excess lax eyelid skin.

Hylaform: Trade name for hyaluronic acid. This injection material provides immediate facial rejuvenation without the necessity for a test dose. It can be repeated every six to nine months.

hyaluronic acid: Generic name for the successor to collagen as the base material in many fillers. It is a natural substance that attracts water in the body. Examples of trade names include Juvéderm, Restylane, Perlane, Hylaform, and Teosyal.

implant: Synthetic material used in reconstruction, such as Goretex for the nose and fixation devices for forehead lifting.

IPL photorejuvenation: IPL (intense pulsed light) is applied to the skin to reduce or eliminate skin imperfections such as birthmarks, small veins, and blemishes.

Juvéderm: Trade name for hyaluronic acid. It is a temporary injected filler used to restore bulk to the face, smooth wrinkles, and plump lips.

laser: Light amplification by stimulated emission of radiation. It is a type of light energy consisting of a focused beam of light at a specific wavelength. It can vaporize the top layer of the skin, making it possible to change facial tissue without making an incision. There are many different types of medical lasers, each having specific treatment applications.

liposuction: A sculpting procedure in which suction and a canula are used to remove fat deposits.

malarplasty: Cheekbone augmentation using implants, fillers, fat, or other materials.

mandible: Lower jaw bone.

maxilla: Upper jaw.

mentoplasty: Surgery to balance a profile by enlarging, reducing, or reshaping the chin.

microdermabrasion: A procedure in which aluminum oxide (bauxite) crystals are sandblasted onto skin to remove old cells to smooth wrinkles, improve pigmentation, and restore "glow."

microsurgery: Surgery done with very small instruments and materials, often assisted with endoscopes or microscopes.

mini- or micro-grafting: Hair-replacement technique in which transplanted pieces of hair-bearing skin or individual hairs are placed to restore hair loss.

mini face-lift: Face-lift with shorter incisions and less skin elevation. It may be useful in younger patients (with less evidence of aging) to achieve a reasonable result with easier recovery.

minimally invasive surgery: Surgery performed through small incisions and/or with minimal tissue trauma. Often assisted with endoscopes.

nasal septum: Cartilage separating the left and right nasal airways.

neuroleptic anesthesia: Anesthesia in which the patient is heavily sedated and free of pain but awake and responsive.

nose job: *See* **rhinoplasty.**

open rhinoplasty: Nasal surgery performed through a small incision between the nostrils, allowing better visualization and treatment, especially in difficult cases. Also called *external rhinoplasty.*

orthognathic surgery: Surgery to correct problems with "bite" or jaw alignment and improve facial contour.

osteotome: A wedge-like instrument used for cutting bone.

otolaryngology: Surgical specialty of the ear, nose, and throat. It involves a wide range of surgery of the head and neck region that includes facial plastic surgery. The specialty is usually called otolaryngology—head and neck surgery.

otoplasty: Surgery to pin back protruding ears.

pedicle: Part of flap left temporarily attached to original site.

Perlane: Trade name for hyaluronic acid.

plastic surgery: Surgery to shape or mold tissues. It can be cosmetic and/or reconstructive. It is the name of the surgical specialty that does plastic surgery of the entire body.

platysma: Either of two broad muscles located on either side of the neck extending from the lower jaw to the clavicle (collarbone).

platysmaplasty: A neck lift, specifically tightening the neck muscles in the midline.

pMMA: Polymethylmethacrylate. It is an inert plastic made in smooth, round microspheres invisible to the naked eye, which act as the filling agent in the permanent filler Artecoll, or Artefill.

ptosis: Drooping.

Restylane: Trade name of hyaluronic acid filler. It is a non-permanent injection product for eliminating tiny lines, enhancing facial contours, and sculpting lips.

rhinoplasty: Cosmetic or reconstructive nasal surgery. It is also known as a *nose job*.

rhytid: Facial wrinkle.

rhytidectomy: Lifting and repositioning of cheek, jaw, and neck skin to reduce signs of aging caused by furrows and sagging of tissues. It is also known as a *face-lift*. The term means "excision of wrinkles."

scalp flap surgery: A hair-replacement method that involves rotating strips of hair-bearing scalp from the side and back of the head to the front and top. It restores the hairline while maintaining normal hair density.

scalp reduction surgery: Surgery to reduce the size of a bald area. It is used to diminish signs of balding and is usually followed by hair transplantation.

septoplasty: Surgical correction of the septum, the part of the nose that divides the right and left nasal cavities, which are often deviated due to trauma and may cause nasal obstruction. It does not usually change nasal appearance.

septorhinoplasty: Cosmetic and/or reconstructive nasal surgery that corrects the nasal septum as well as the appearance of the nose.

sclerotherapy: Injection of veins, usually with saline, to decrease their appearance.

skin-muscle flap blepharoplasty: Lower eyelid lift done through a fine incision made externally just beneath the eyelashes.

Silastic: A firm implant popular for chin, cheek, and nasal augmentation.

SMAS: Superficial musculoaponeurotic system. It is a layer of fascia beneath the facial skin that envelops the muscles and translates muscle action into facial expressions. It is frequently modified and used to lift the face in the face-lift.

SMAS face-lift: *See* **standard face-lift.**

SPF: Sun protection factor. It is the measured amount of sun protection a sunblock provides. For example, SPF 30 means that you can spend thirty times as much time in the sun to get the same sun exposure as you would without the sunblock.

standard face-lift: A routine face-lift with elevation of skin, lifting of the fascia underneath, and removal of excess, lax skin.

submentoplasty: Suctioning the pocket of accumulated fat under the chin and sculpting the neck muscles through a small incision beneath the chin. It is usually done in conjunction with a face-lift.

sun protection factor: *See* **SPF.**

trade name: The name created by a company to identify a particular drug. It often has some similarity to the generic name. For example, Juvéderm is a trade name.

transconjunctival blepharoplasty: An eyelid lift done through an incision behind the lower eyelid, removing bags but leaving no external incision.

trichophytic forehead lift: A forehead lift in which the incision is made along the top of the forehead at the hairline.

twilight sleep: *See* **neuroleptic anesthesia.**

wattle: Sagging neck skin in the midline, usually due to excess skin and fat.

APPENDIX

COSMETIC SURGERY SPECIALISTS

Several different types of specialists may provide excellent cosmetic facial surgery and treatments.

Facial Plastic Surgeons

Most facial plastic surgeons have done specialty training in otolaryngology—head and neck surgery and/or plastic surgery. They tend to specialize in facial work alone. Those with additional training or experience may be certified by the American Board of Facial Plastic and Reconstructive Surgery (ABFPRS).

Plastic Surgeons

Most plastic surgeons are trained in plastic surgery. Some, however, are "double-boarded," meaning that they also trained in otolaryngology—head and neck surgery. These specialists may operate in all areas of plastic surgery, including hand surgery, bone surgery, body cosmetic surgery, cosmetic facial surgery, and more. Some will specialize in cosmetic facial surgery, others may do other parts of the body, and some may do no cosmetic facial surgery.

Ophthalmologists

Ophthalmologists are surgically trained and may specialize in oculoplastic surgery or plastic surgery around the eye. Many of these surgeons do reconstructive and cosmetic eyelid surgery but tend not to do other cosmetic facial surgery.

Dermatologists

Dermatologists are trained through the internal medicine route, as opposed to the surgical specialty route. Some specialize in dermatologic surgery. These surgeons reconstruct cancer surgical defects and may perform a large number of cosmetic treatments, including facial fillers, Botox, etc. Some do body liposuction.

Oral (Maxillofacial) Surgeons

Oral (or maxillofacial) surgeons are trained through the dental school route as opposed to the medical school route. In the United States, many dental schools now combine their training with medical schools. Their graduates have combined M.D. and D.D.S. (doctor of dental surgery) degrees. These surgeons specialize in advanced upper and lower jaw surgery, often in conjunction with orthodontic treatment, to correct facial deformities for both cosmetic and reconstructive purposes.

DOCTOR CREDENTIALS

Most physicians have undergraduate degrees, such as a bachelor of science (B.Sc.) or bachelor of arts (B.A.), but usually don't list them, as they have so many other degrees. The doctor of medicine (M.D.) is the most common, though some foreign schools have other names, such as M.B.B.S. in the United Kingdom. In the United States, some doctors complete their medical training as Doctors of Osteopathy (D.O.).

These credentials indicate that you're a physician and surgeon who, theoretically, can practice internal medicine, basic surgery, psychiatry, obstetrics and gynecology, pediatrics, etc. across the full breadth of the medical spectrum. General or family practitioners usually have a broad rather than deep knowledge of medicine. They're very much the gatekeepers to more specialized care. They're invaluable in carrying out primary care and making appropriate referrals. Today, many complete a two- or three-year family practice training program and are certified.

With medical or surgical specialty training, after four years or more of post-M.D. training, you become "board eligible." This means that your training program director confirms that you've satisfactorily completed the training program and are eligible to sit the "board," "certification" or "fellowship" examinations. These are all more or less equivalent terms for the defining specialty credential that confirms your level of competence to practice independently and to apply for hospital privileges in your area of training.

In the United States, the physician or surgeon can usually apply for and receive a state medical licence to practice in his or her specialty as "board eligible" in that specialty. In Canada, a surgeon can't practice by simply completing the training program but must also pass a credentialing examination through the Royal College of Physicians and Surgeons of Canada to obtain his or her F.R.C.S.C. (Fellow of the Royal College of Surgeons of Canada). Most medical and surgical specialists in the Commonwealth countries take these exams. They consist of both written and oral exams over one or two days, testing the full gamut of the specialty.

Surgeons who go on to do even further superspecialty training, such as facial plastic surgery, are said to be doing a fellowship. They can describe themselves as "fellowship trained" in their superspecialties or board-certified in the name of the specialty board (for example, the American Board of Facial Plastic and Reconstructive Surgery).

MEDICAL ORGANIZATIONS

Most physicians with appropriate training in performing cosmetic surgery belong to one or more medical organizations that recognize them and protect the public interest. They also promote the surgeons' educational and other socioeconomic interests.

Certifying or Credentialing Boards and Colleges

Universities that provide medical school training bestow the doctor of medicine (M.D.) degree. In the United States, this may include osteopathic colleges. There's a separate federal or national board that examines candidates and makes them "board-certified" in the United States or "Fellow of the Royal College of Surgeons" in Canada.

In the U.S. and Canada, the American Board of Facial Plastic and Reconstructive Surgery (ABFPRS) certifies surgeons who have completed the additional one-year fellowship training and requirements beyond those for certification in plastic surgery and otolaryngology—head and neck surgery. The successful candidate is then a diplomate of the ABFPRS. Some surgeons practice for at least five years and then sit the examinations.

Many boards belong to national groups, such as the American Board of Medical Specialties in the United States and the Royal College of Physicians and Surgeons in Canada. However, other boards that aren't members of either group may be recognized as having similar requirements (e.g., the American Board of Facial Plastic and Reconstructive Surgery).

Regulatory or Licensing Boards

A surgeon or physician can't begin practice upon receiving an M.D. or specialty degree. He or she must first obtain a state or provincial licence. Boards or colleges in various jurisdictions review the applicant's training and malpractice or complaint history, obtain reference letters, and follow other criteria prior to granting a licence to practice medicine.

These boards or colleges receive patient complaints and mete out suspensions or other penalties for practice that falls below the expected standard of care. They exist to protect the public and serve the profession.

Specialty certifying or credentialing boards usually do background checks with these regulatory or licensing boards prior to bestowing their "board-certified" distinction. They can suspend or rescind a surgeon's certification for unprofessional conduct.

Academies and Associations

The American Medical Association (AMA) and Canadian Medical Association (CMA) embrace the majority of practicing physicians and surgeons. They represent the political and socioeconomic interests of physicians and surgeons, and take a major role in educating the public about medicine. They promote health care public policy.

Most specialities have their own academies that provide continuing medical education courses, represent the specific interests of their membership to the public, and inform the public about the work of their specialists. These include the American Academy of Facial Plastic and Reconstructive Surgery (AAFPRS), the Canadian Academy of Facial Plastic and Reconstructive Surgery (CAFPRS), the American

Society of Plastic and Reconstructive Surgery (ASPRS), the American Society of Aesthetic Plastic Surgery (ASAPS), and the Canadian Society for Aesthetic Plastic Surgery (CSAPS).

Foundations

Many specialty academies and associations have foundations, tax-exempt arms of the organizations that are responsible for education, research, and humanitarian work. For example, the Education and Research Foundation of the American Academy of Facial Plastic and Reconstructive Surgery supports the FACE TO FACE humanitarian missions overseas and the domestic violence project in the United States to assist women who have suffered facial trauma as a result of domestic violence. Other foundations, such as the Canadian Foundation for Facial Plastic and Reconstructive Surgery, are established for humanitarian purposes alone, usually with very specific goals and programs.

BIBLIOGRAPHY

Alam, M., and Dover, J.S. "On Beauty: Evolution, Psychosocial Considerations, and Surgical Enhancement." *Archives of Dermatology* 137 (June 2001): 795–807.

Alsarraf, R., Larrabee, W.F., Anderson, F., Murakami, C.S., and Johnson, C.M. "Measuring Cosmetic Facial Plastic Surgery Outcomes: A Pilot Study." *Archfacial Plastic Surgery Outcomes* 1 (July–September 2003).

Bransford, Helen. *Welcome to Your Face-lift*. New York: Doubleday, 1997.

Ciaschini, M., and Bernard, S.L. *History of Plastic Surgery*. Retrieved January 2005, from http://www.emedicine.com.

Etcoff, Nancy. *Survival of the Prettiest: The Science of Beauty*. New York: Doubleday, 1999.

Goin, John, and Kraft Goin, Marcia. *Changing the Body: Psychological Effects of Plastic Surgery*. London: Williams & Wilkins, 1981.

Gladwell, Malcolm. *Blink: The Power of Thinking Without Thinking*. New York: Little, Brown and Company, 2005.

Gladwell, Malcolm. *The Tipping Point: How Little Things Can Make a Big Difference*. New York: Little, Brown and Company, 2002.

Glaser, Gabrielle. *The Nose: A Profile of Sex, Beauty and Survival*. New York: Atria Books, 2002.

Konner, Melvin. *The Tangled Wing: Biological Constraints on the Human Spirit*, 2nd edition. New York: Henry Holt and Company, 2002.

Litner, J.A., Rotenberg, B.W., Dennis, M., and Adamson, P.A. "Impact of cosmetic facial surgery on satisfaction with appearance and quality of life." *Archives of Facial Plastic Surgery* 10, no. 2 (March/April 2008): 79–83.

Lorenc, Z. Paul, and Hall, Trish. *A Little Work: Behind the Doors of a Park Avenue Plastic Surgeon.* New York: St. Martin's Press, 2004.

McNeill, Daniel. *The Face: A Natural History.* New York: Little, Brown and Company, 1998.

Muley, Gunakar. "Plastic Surgery in Ancient India." Retrieved January 2009, from http://www.vigyanpraser.gov.in.

Pease, Allan, and Pease, Barbara. *Why Men Don't Listen and Women Can't Read Maps.* New York: Broadway Books, 2000.

Penton-Voak, I.S., and Perrett, D.I. "Consistency and individual differences in facial attractiveness judgements—an evolutionary perspective." *Social Research* 67 (March 2000): 219–245.

Rana, R.E., and Arora, B.S. "History of Plastic Surgery in India." *Journal of Postgraduate Medicine* 48 (2002): 76–78.

Rivers, Joan, and Frankel, Valerie. *Men Are Stupid . . . And They Like Big Boobs: A Woman's Guide to Beauty Through Plastic Surgery.* New York: Simon and Shuster, 2008.

Rodgers, Joann Ellison. *Sex: A Natural History.* New York: Henry Holt and Company, 2001.

Scharff, J., and Levy, Jaedene. *The Face-lift Diaries: What It's Really Like to Have a Face-lift.* Charleston: BookSurge, 2004.

ABOUT THE AUTHOR

Dr. Peter Adamson is a facial plastic surgeon who has had a successful and respected practice in Toronto, Ontario, since 1981. He is certified by the Royal College of Physicians and Surgeons of Canada in Otolaryngology—Head and Neck Surgery. He is board-certified by the American Board of Otolaryngology and is a Fellow of the American College of Surgeons. Dr. Adamson is also board-certified by the American Board of Facial Plastic and Reconstructive Surgery. He is a professor and head of the Division of Facial Plastic and Reconstructive Surgery, Department of Otolaryngology—Head and Neck Surgery, at the University of Toronto and a staff surgeon at the Toronto General Hospital.

Dr. Adamson is widely published and regularly lectures to national and international audiences on his specialty. He is a member and has been president of both the Canadian and American Academies of Facial Plastic and Reconstructive Surgery. He is past president and senior advisor to the American Board of Facial Plastic and Reconstructive Surgery.

Dr. Adamson is also president of the Canadian Foundation for Facial Plastic Surgery, a Toronto-based not-for-profit organization that supports international humanitarian medical missions, such as FACE TO FACE. Funds are directed to help cover travel and accommodation costs of mission surgeons who donate their time and skills to help disfigured children in less fortunate countries reclaim their lives. Visit www.thecanadianfoundation.com for more information about the organization and the causes supported through donations.

Dr. Adamson is donating 10 percent of the proceeds from the sale of *Fabulous Faces* to the Canadian Foundation for Facial Plastic and Reconstructive Surgery to support its humanitarian missions.

INDEX